I0422186

The Benefits of Nature
Natural Skin Care Guide
Alana Monet-Telfer

Introduction

Everywhere in the beauty market there are many products being sold which state that they can help clear your skin, remove dirt, remove oil, rid free radicals, retain moisture, bring back moisture, and overall give you young and youthful skin. I was one of the unfortunate people who believed the hype and brought every type of new beauty scrub, mask, and skin treatment possible. Unfortunately, none of them worked for my skin, and I thought I would have spotty, dry, and dirty looking skin forever. I was in this pit of despair until the age of fifteen when I started researching and finding beauty skin therapies which used natural foods. Therefore, once I started using these recipes, I realised that there are a lot more benefits of food on skin; than the products used in the market which contain chemicals which caused skin to be damaged and unhealthy. This is the man reason why the book was created; as I know how hard it can be to defend our skin from the daily elements; while being fooled with these products which claim they would help and skin; and in the end only give us financial problems and holes in our pockets.

Aim

After three years of using natural beauty skin therapy treatments, I have decided to turn this into a project; therefore, by doing this I'll be able to help others solve their skin problems and insecurities.

Warnings: In this book I shall give warning notes which explain the possible hazards of the skin care masks and which types of skin certain masks would not be advisable for. The warning notes will be in red.

Organic Foods: Although I am not able to get every single skin recipe to be organic, it's still vital to use organic foods. The use of non organic foods can be risky; since some will contain pesticides and chemicals from farming and growing; and I am sure nobody would want farm chemicals and pesticides absorbing into the skin and cause damage from the inside out. If you are unable to get organic foods for your recipes; it is still ok to use food from the store.

Hazards: The only hazards that will come from these recipes are that they go into you eyes; or they can cause allergic reactions. If the mask goes into you eye; use cold water to rinse it off immediately. If you get an allergic reaction, get help immediately.

For People with Food Allergies: If you have any allergies to any of the foods used in the mask recipes; its best to not use the food you are allergic to. You might not get the benefits of the food you're allergic to; however, you will still get the benefits of the other foods which will give you clean, spotless, and clear skin.

Fact: Do you know that 23% of the cause of ageing and skin problems comes naturally from our bodies? Therefore, this means that the 77% of the causes of skin ageing and problems comes from the environment. If we can learn how to combat the 77% using the benefits of nature and its goods; you can finally have the skin you have always wanted and dreamed of.

After Care Skin Treatment
What do I use as my After Care Treatment?
After using any of the masks listed in this book; my skin feels the benefits, however, without some type of after skin treatment, my skin would become dry and even more damaged then before. The reason for this is because the natural oils of my skin would have been taken along with the dirt and bacteria. This means that my body is creating new natural oils to replenish the skin. In order to help the skin with this process, as well as help my skin to be moisturised and avoid skin damage from the after affect of the masks; I use my after treatment face cream, lip balm, and eye cream. The brand of after treatment products comes from the brand called Simple. Another skin care treatment I use for my skin is Palmers Coconut Butter Formula with Vitamin E.

Why do I Use Simple Skin Care Products?
Simple is a special skin care product which helps people with sensitive skin to have soft and glowing skin which looks unaffected by our environment. Although my skin is not too sensitive (its combination type skin I still use this product because it is pure and doesn't contain any the of chemicals, fragrances, or colourings which other products have in their face cream, lip balm, and eye creams. I used to use Nivea skin care face creams, however, I found that they contained chemicals which did worse damage to the skin then our environment, and therefore, I ditched it and looked for a pure skin care product until I came across Simple. For me I use Simple Rich Moisturiser since I usually suffer from dry skin, however, the product you use depending on your skin and how it reacts after its been treated with a mask.

Why do I use Palmers Coconut Butter Formula with Vitamin E?
Using this Coco Butter after a mask (especially masks that take a lot of old and natural oils out of the skin) helps the skin to be re-moisturised and plump up again. After doing any mask, apply this butter formula to your face and sleep with it on overnight. Once morning comes, wash the butter off with a scrub followed by warm water. After you face has been rinsed you should have plump smooth and youthful skin. For people who have outbreaks from too much oil, or have oily skin, this is not recommended. The application of this butter over a period of time stops premature ageing and keeps skin smooth and soft.

What does Simple Skin care do for my Skin?

Simple Rich Moisturiser face cream helps new oils to replenish and moisturise my skin. After I've used any of my facial masks, and apply the face cream on my face, my skin feels smooth and soft; just as if I had baby skin again.

Benefits of Nature Skin care Recipes

Apple

Although I don't like apples (because they make me sick if I eat them) I still know that apples have wonderful benefits for the skin. After testing apple on skin to see the many benefits of skin; I was able to find the benefits, therefore, the benefits of apples on skin are:

- **Treatment for Acne:** Using Apple Cider vinegar on the skin has been proven to rid skin of bacteria, oils, and balance the skins pH level. By the apple cider vinegar working on the skin, this combats the symptoms and problems of acne.
- **Treatment for Blemishes:** Apple cider vinegar is also great for removing overnight blemishes.
- **Sunburn Treatment:** Apple skin contains phenols which give UV-B protection against the rays of the sun. The apples that are high in these phenols are Braeburn, Fuji, and Red Delicious Apples from Granny Smiths.
- **De-ageing treatment:** Granny Smiths Red Delicious Apples aid in the fortifying of collagen and elastin. This leaves your skin tight in elasticity and youthful in looks. Consumption of apples also helps reduce find wrinkles and lines.
- **Skin Toner:** The nutrients and antioxidants in apples help to tone and even skin.
- **Eye Treatment:** By putting slices of apples over the eyes; this stops, or reduces, puffiness.
- **Hydrating:** Since apple contains a lot of water, blending it and applying it to your face hydrates dull and de-hydrated skin.
- **Cooling and Exfoliating:** While researching apple mask recipes I came across another benefits which I didn't know about, therefore, apple helps to cool and exfoliate dead cells of the skin. The information below explains this benefit in more detail:

Apples have a very cooling, slightly exfoliating effect on our skin due to the mild acids in the fruit. When applied to the skin, apples bring circulation and nourishment to the skin.

(Taken from http://www.epicbeautyguide.com)

Recipes that Use Apple

1. **Apple Mask for Smooth Moist Skin:** Mash up 1/2 of an apple — include the skin, but do *not* include the core or seeds. You can also mash it up with a mortar and pestle, or in a food processor.   In a small dish, mix the mashed apple with 1 Tbsp. raw honey. (Optional: also add your 1 egg yolk). Apply and leave on 10–20 minutes. Rinse off with warm water. Finish with a splash of cool water. You may then tone with a floral water (hydrosol), quality natural toner like Sophyto or 100% Pure, or (my favorite) neem leaf extract spray. Follow up with a natural moisturizer or gently massage in a few drops of organic extra virgin olive oil.

2. **Mask Treatment for Acne:** Try the apple zinger face mask for reducing acne if you have oily skin. Finely grate one medium peeled apple and combine it with 5 tbsp. of honey. Apply the face mask to your skin and leave in on for 10 minutes. Rinse with cool water. Add uncooked oatmeal to exfoliate if you have combination skin.

3. **Mask Treatment for Oily Skin:** Start a savory apple face mask by cutting up one ripe peeled apple, setting aside the core and seeds. Cut the apple into large cubes and place in your food processor or blender and pulse until the fruit is pureed. Thoroughly mix the fruit with 2 tbsp. honey and 1 tsp. sage, and then refrigerate for 10 minutes. While the fruit mask is chilling, you can prepare your skin by either steaming it or washing it. Apply the face mask and let it dry for approximately 20 minutes, then gently peel off the mask or remove it with water. This mask is best for oily skin, and has a unique scent because of the sage.

4. **Exfoliating Apple Mask:** Make the Aphrodite face mask by combining 1 tbsp. applesauce with 1 tbsp. wheat germ until they form a paste and then apply to a clean face. Allow the face pack to dry completely and then gently remove with water and a soft cloth. Using cool water to wash your face will help to close your pores. The wheat germ can also aid in exfoliating the skin. Add 1 tsp. of cinnamon to make an autumn-scented mask.

Avocado

This fruit is known as one of the most moisturising fruits which give skin the right balance in oils. The avocado also has other names, for example, Persea gratissima or P. americana, Avocado, Avocado, Alligator pear, Avocado pear, Fuerte, Gwen, Hass, Pinkerton, Reed, Zutano, Aguacate, Avocat, Abacate, and Ahuacatl. Other benefits of avocado on skin are:

- **Cleanses Skin:** Avocados are rich in vitamin A, hence, this is useful for removing dead skin cells. Another way avocado cleanses skin is that the amino acids in them (called Glutamine) protects the skin against sun damage.

- **Skin Softener:** One of the things I have found when I use avocado in my masks, or hair, is that it deeply penetrates the skin and restores nutrients to it. Avocados are especially good for people who suffer from dry skin.

- **Skin Renewal:** Avocado helps with skin renewal and blood circulation to the skin.

- **Anti Ageing properties:** Avocado contains antioxidants which help reduce wrinkles and other symptoms of ageing. They are able to do this by getting rid of toxins which are on the surface of the skin.

- **Hair Treatment:** This use of avocado in hair causes the pores of the skin to be deeply penetrates with nutrients. It also aids dry, brittle, and damaged hair. Avocado can also make hair shiny; due to the vitamin E contained in it.

Recipes that use Avocado

1. **Avocado Body Moisturiser:** To make your own body moisturizer simply mash 1 or 2 avocados and add honey or your favourite essential oil. Apply the avocado to your skin and leave on for 20 to 30 minutes before rinsing with warm water.

2. **Anti-ageing Avocado Mask:** Applying 1 mashed avocado as a facial mask and leaving it on for about 20 minutes before rinsing will help to remove these toxins.

3. **Hair Treatment:** Simply massage the avocado and egg mixture into your hair and scalp and leave in for about 20 minutes. Then wash and condition with your regular shampoo and conditioner.

4. **Hair Treatment Conditioner:** To a blender add half a cup of Extra Virgin Olive Oil, Coconut oil, Honey, shop brought hair conditioner of you choice, two table spoons of lime, Lemon (Or both) juice and a whole avocado. Blend it all together until there is a thick consistency. Leave it in the hair over night, detangle, and rinse hair with Luke warm water.

5. **Avocado Mask for Dehydrated Skin:** Add avocado and pineapple chunks to a food processor. Squeeze the lime to extract juice and pulp onto the mixture. Process until smooth, but textured. Add olive oil and honey and mix with a fork until well blended.

6. **Avocado Mask for Moisturising:** In shallow bowl, mash avocado until smooth; add yogurt and honey; stir until combined. Apply evenly to face and cover eyes with cucumber slices; put on your favourite tunes, lie back and allow mask to set for 15 minutes; rinse with warm water.

7. **Avocado Mask for Oily Skin:** In blender, combine avocado, egg white and lemon juice; whirl until smooth. Apply evenly to face; leave on 20 minutes while you phone your best friend and play catch up; rinse with warm water.

8. **Avocado, Lemon, Cumber, and Lime Mask:** To a bowl combine half of an avocado, 2two tablespoons of Lemon, two tablespoons of lime juice, and a quarter of a cucumber. Make sure the cucumber has had its skin peeled off before combining it with the other ingredients. Once you have the mask apply it to face, leave on for forty minutes before rinsing the mask off with semi warm water.

Banana

Bananas are very important fruit, not only because of their health benefits to the body but also to the skin. The information below explains abit about the origin of Bananas.

Edible bananas originated in the Indo-Malaysian region reaching to northern Australia. They were known only by hearsay in the Mediterranean region in the 3rd Century B.C., and are believed to have been first carried to Europe in the 10th Century A.D. Early in the 16th Century, Portuguese mariners transported the plant from the West African coast to South America. The types found in cultivation in the Pacific have been traced to eastern Indonesia from where they spread to the Marquesas and by stages to Hawaii.

(Taken from www.hort.purdue.edu)

The benefits that Banana has on skin are:

+ **Nutrition's Skin:** Banana contains nutrients which are very important to the skin. For example, banana contains Vitamin C which aids in the integrity of the skin and produces collagen in the body.

+ **Antioxidant:** Banana contains antioxidants which protects the skin from free radical and oxygen damage. Banana also contains another free radical fighting agent called manganese.

+ **De-ageing:** The consumption, or use, of Banana can reduce signs of ageing and possible hair loss.

+ **Hydrating:** A Banana contains 75% of water by weight, hence, this helps hydrate the skin, since the skin will absorb all the water.

+ **Gives Healthy Skin:** Banana keeps the skin glowing and healthy, hence, this is due to the vitamin B6 (or Pyridoxine) which it has.

Recipes that use Banana

1. **Banana Mask for Oily Skin:** Mash up the banana, then mix in the honey. For best results, put the ingredients in a blender. Add a few drops of juice from an orange or a lemon. Apply to face for 15 minutes before rinsing with a cool washcloth or a steaming warm washcloth. Follow with your regular moisturizer.

2. **Banana Mask for oily Skin Second Treatment:** Mix together half a masked Banana, one table spoon of honey, and one tablespoon of yogurt

together. Apply the mixture to face and leave it on for 5-10 minutes before rinsing your face off with semi warm water.

3. **Avocado and Banana Mask:** Mix half an avocado and half of a banana together. Apply to face, leave it on for fifteen minutes, and rinse face off with luke warm water.

4. **Banana Face Mask:** Mash half of a banana, apply to your face, leave on for 5 minutes, before rinsing your face off with luke warm water.

5. **Banana and Honey Face Mask:** Mix half a banana together with a tablespoon of honey. Apply to face, leave the mask on until dry, and finally rinse your face off with semi-warm water.

6. **Banana Mask for Acne:** Combine 1 whole banana, one tablespoon of honey and a teaspoon of lemon juice. Apply to face, leave on for fifteen minutes, before rinsing the mask off with semi-warm water.

7. **Banana Mask for Dry Skin:** To a bowl combine half a masked banana, half a cup of oatmeal, one tablespoon of honey, and one egg yolk. Once you have the mixture, apply the mask to the face; leave it on for fifteen minutes, before finally rinsing the mask off with semi-warm water.

8. **De-ageing Banana Mask:** Mix half of a mashed banana, one tablespoon of honey, and 1 egg yolk together. Once you have done this apply the mixture to your face, leave it on for 30-40 minutes, and rinse the mask off using semi warm water.

9. **Banana and Milk Mask:** Mix together half of a mashed banana, one tablespoon of honey, and one tablespoon of milk. Apply mixture to your face, Leave on for 15, and Rise off with cool water.

10. **Banana and Oatmeal Face Mask:** Combine half a cup of oatmeal, 1 table spoon of honey, 1 egg yolk and half a mashed banana. Apply mixture to your face, Leave on for 15, and Rise off with cool water.

Baking Soda
Baking soda is used in many ingredients, especially baking. However, baking soda can be good for the skin too, hence, the benefits of baking soda on the skin are:

1. **Closes pores**: Baking soda helps to close pores, which stops dirt, oil, and residue for building up inside of the pores.

2. **Make up remover**: It's especially useful for removing make up.

3. **Exfoliate**: removes dead skin cells.

4. **Leaves skin smooth**.

5. **Inflammation**: Treats inflammation from sunburns.

6. **Treats Acne**: Acne is caused when excessive sebum is produced, blocking the skin's pores and allowing bacteria to get trapped within. The body's immune system attacks the bacteria leaving the skin around the area inflamed. According to UBeautyPortal.com, bacteria require an acidic setting to multiply. The alkaline nature of baking soda prevents this from happening.

7. **Oil Absorber:** Baking soda also helps keeps pores open and absorbs excess oil from the skin.

Recipes Using Baking Soda

1. **Baking Soda Black Head Scrub:** Mix one tablespoon of granulated sugar, one tablespoon of baking soda, and two tablespoons of water together. Apply to skin, massage into skin for three minutes before rinsing your face off with luke warm water.

2. **Baking Soda Oatmeal face mask:** Make a paste of these ingredients: 1 Tbsp Baking Soda, 2 Tbsp Oatmeal, and one tsp of Honey. Add water if required. Slather a layer this mask on your face for 15 mins. Wash off with warm water.

3. **Baking Soda Orange soda mask:** Mix Soda into the Orange juice till it is completely dissolved. Apply this juice on face and neck, massage in circular movements after 10 mins. This is an instant skin brightener.

Warning: Always use moisturiser on you face after using these masks. Baking soda cleans the pores, but can be very draying for the skin afterwards, hence, it's very important to use a rich moisturiser for the face. If you have any allergic reactions to baking soda, do not use these mask recipes. Baking soda should not be over used on the face, since this can lead to patchy skin, dryness, and skin bleaches; which can make the skin on your face brighter than the natural colour of your skin on your body.

Castor Oil

Castor oil is known to have medical and curative uses; hence, this is why castor oil, anthology very thick and oily, is a great benefit for the skin. The benefits of castor oil on the skin are:

- **Cures Acne:** Castor oil surprisingly contains a ricinoleic acid which kills any viruses or bacteria that are on the skin or deep in the skin pores. This means the castor oil to penetrate deep into the skin tissue.

- **Smoothes skin:** Because of the castor oils deep penetration properties (since it's the only oil that can penetrate deep into skin), it's great for keeping skin smooth and youthful.

- **Cures Scars:** The deep penetration of castor oil can help loosen internal and external dead skin tissue from scars.

- **Cure for Stretch Marks.**

- **Aid for Eyes Lashes and Eyebrows:** Adding a little castor oil over the eyes lashes helps thicken and strengthen eye lashes.

Recipes that Use Castor Oil

1. **Aid for other Skin Treatments:** It can be used in conjunction with other skin recipes to help benefit the overall skin.

2. **Castor oil for scars:** place castor oil on a scar and leave it on there for one-two hours each day.

3. **Castor Oil for Acne:**

   To treat acne, dab a hot damp washcloth all over your face in the evening before you go to bed. The heat will gently open the pores on your face. After this, massage a little castor oil gently into the skin. Leave on overnight. Repeat this daily for 1 to 2 weeks to see results. You can also repeat this twice in the day, once at night and once in the morning.

(Taken From http://skinverse.com/castor-oils-many-uses-for-beautiful-skin-and-hair.html#Castoroilacne)

4. **Castor Oil Cleanser:** You can rub castor oil over you face to cleanse it. You don't need a lot of this oil, since it's very thick. Apply the castor onto the face; leave it on for an hour, before rinsing the oil away with luke warm to cold water.

Warning: Using Castor oil over excessively (meaning using castor oil in every single mask you make or 24/7) can cause the skin to become lose for 1-2 weeks. Although this is temporary, the risk can be avoided by using other natural skin recipes as well as taking a break from using castor oil for awhile.

Cucumber

Cucumber is another great vegetable. The information below explains abit about the cucumber:

Cucumber is a vegetable that belongs to the same family as pumpkins, zucchinis and other squashes. It has a dark green skin, which reveals whitish or very light green flesh, when peeled. There are basically two types of cucumbers - the pickling varieties and the slicing varieties. Of these, the pickling variety is relatively small, around 2 - 4 inches long.
(Taken from www.articlesbase.com)

The benefits of cucumber (or its scientific name known as Cucumis Sativus) are:

- **Combats eye swelling:** Cucumber deals with the problem of eye swelling. The reason for this is due to the cucumbers high silica content.
- **Combats Sunburn.**
- **Water Retention Solution:** Cucumber contains ascorbic and caffeic acids, therefore, this deals with water retention in the body as well as eye swelling.
- **Skin Softener:** Skin and Cucumber share the same level of Hydrogen, therefore, this is good because it helps to cleanse and make the skin soft and supple.

Recipes that Use Cucumber

1. **Cucumber Mask for Soft Skin:** Blend 4 - 5 leafs of fresh mint, Peel, and de-seeds the cucumber. After doing this add mint leaves to the cucumber to make a puree. Beat egg white and keep it separate, then add this egg white to the cucumber mixture. Apply this evenly on your face for 20 minutes and then rinse it with water and pat it dry.

2. **Yogurt Cucumber Mask:** Peel and cut the cucumber into small cubes, you can remove the seeds for a smoother consistency of the mask. Put it in a food processor and add half of the yogurt and the teaspoon of milk powder. Blend it until you have a smooth substance that will stay on your face without running. Don't overdo the blending. Spread the paste gently and equally with your fingertips on your clean face and neck: keep the eye area clear. Now lie down, relax and leave the mask on for 10-15 minutes. Finally wash it off with a warm wash cloth and warm water and end with a splash of cold; pat your skin dry with a clean towel.

3. **Aloe Vera Cucumber Mask**: Peel half of the cucumber and cut it in pieces. Put the cucumber pieces together with the two tablespoons of aloe vera in a food processor and blend them until you have a nice smooth paste. Spread the paste gently and equally with your fingertips on your clean face and neck: keep the eye area clear. Now lie down, relax and leave the mask on for 30 minutes. Finally wash it off with cold water; pat your skin dry with a clean towel.

4. **Almond Butter Cucumber Mask:** Peel quarter of a cucumber, take out the seeds, cut it in small pieces and put it in a blender. Mash it until it is nice and watery, it should be cucumber juice. Now mix this thoroughly together with the one tablespoon of almond butter. Spread the paste gently and equally with a facial mask brush or spatula on your clean face and neck: keep the eye area clear. Now lie down, relax and leave the mask on for 5-10 minutes. Then wash it off with lukewarm water; pat your skin dry with a clean towel.

5. **Honey, Lemon, Banana, and Cucumber Mask:** Warm up the table spoon of honey until it becomes liquid (not too hot) by putting it in a small glass or metal bowl which is immersed in hot water. Put half of the banana and half of the cucumber in a food processor and mash them. Add the liquid honey, four tablespoons of lemon juice and mix until you have a smooth workable substance. Spread the paste gently and equally with your fingertips on your clean face and neck: keep the eye area clear. Now lie down, relax and leave the mask on for 30 minutes. Then wash it off with lukewarm water; pat your skin dry with a clean towel. Finally apply a moisturizer, this way you "seal" your skin to keep the water inside.

6. **Honey, Yogurt, Oatmeal, and Cucumber Mask:** Warm up the two tablespoons of honey until it becomes liquid (not too hot) by putting it in a small glass or metal bowl which is immersed in hot water. Peel the cucumber and cut it into cubes. Put this together with the liquid honey, yogurt and oatmeal in a blender. Mix until you have a paste that is consistent enough so it will stay on your face without running. Spread the paste gently and equally with a facial mask brush or spatula on your clean face and neck: keep the eye area clear. Now lie down, relax and leave the mask on for 30 minutes. Then wash it off with lukewarm water; pat your skin dry with a clean towel. Finally apply a moisturizer, this way you "seal" your skin to keep the water inside

Cinnamon

Cinnamon is a spice which is made from the grinding down of the Evergreen tree in the rainy season; therefore, the reason for this is because in the rainy season the bark is soft and flexible. With Cinnamons woody, mild, and striking flavour, it is known as one of the most used spices in the world.

Benefits of Cinnamon on Skin
The benefits that come from cinnamon when it's used on skin are:

- **Smoothes and Plumps Skin:** When cinnamon is used on skin, it causes blood from the body to rise to the surface of the skin; therefore, this will cause a swelling and plumping which will make your skin, or face, smooth, plump, and moisturised.
- **Cleanser:** Cinnamon reacts as an exfoliate to nourish hair follicles.
- **Eczema Treatment**: Using one tablespoon of honey and 1 table spoon of cinnamon can rid patches of Eczema once it's applied to the affected areas.
- **Acne Treatment:** Since Cinnamon brings blood and oxygen to the skin; this helps fight acne. The use of Cinnamon on acne skin causes dryness, therefore, this stops acne spreading.

Recipes that Use Cinnamon
1. **Cinnamon and Nutmeg Face Scrub:** This helps with bringing blood and oxygen to the surface of the skin; therefore, your skin will feel soft and look plump. To make this mixture mix once table spoon of honey with one table spoon of Cinnamon and Nutmeg. Use this as a face scrub and exfoliate your face for about two minutes before rinsing it off with slightly cold water.
2. **Cinnamon, Nutmeg, and Lemon Face Scrub:** This face scrub is similar to the Lemon and Lime skin peel mask, however, this scrub is a quicker way to remove a layer of dead skin; as to the Lemon and Lime mask which needs about 40 minutes to work. For this beauty scrub mix one tablespoon of Cinnamon, one table spoon of Nutmeg, and two table spoons of lemon (or lime) juice. Once the mixture is ready, scrub your face gently with it and leave it to work on the skin for eight seconds. Rinse face as usual with cold water.

Warning: Do not leave this scrub on your face for more than ten seconds. If you leave it on for more than ten seconds it will cause burning and skin damage; due to the mask taking off too much of the skin at once. People who suffer from severe dry skin should not use this.

Warning 2: Do not use too much cinnamon, followed by nutmeg on your face. This caused extreme burning and severe skin damage. If this happens, use yogurt on your face for a week to repair and moisturise the skin.

Chocolate

13

For everybody chocolate gives them different emotions and feelings. For example; it can make one feel happy, make one feel in love (due to the endorphins in chocolate), or help one to relax after a busy and sometimes even stressful day. What people might not know is that chocolate is good for skin, therefore, its can give great benefits and help your skin to be radical free and healthy. The benefits of chocolate on skin are:

- **Irritated Skin Treatment:** For people with irritated skin; chocolate can help to sooth and calm it.
- **Blood Circulator:** Just as Cinnamon and Nutmeg bring the blood to the surface of the skin (Which helps increase blood circulation around the body); Chocolate also can do that too. This is good for people who are allergic to Cinnamon and Nutmeg but still want the same benefits.
- **Uv Protector:** In dark chocolate the flavonnoids protect skin from the presence of UV ray light from the sun. This decreases the chance of sun burn and skin cancer.
- **Skin Softener:** Chocolate contains skin softening properties due to chocolate containing coco butter. It's also very moisturising.
- **De ageing treatment:** It can smooth out wrinkles because if its anti-oxidant properties. It also helps to protect elastin (Elasticity of the skin), and collagen.
- **Nutrition:** Chocolate contains nutrients which nourish the skin.
- **Skin Renewal:** Chocolate, when applied to skin, can remove dead skin cells and speed of the process of cell renewal
- **Hydration:** Properties of the chocolate help to hydrate the skin.

Recipes that use Chocolate
- ❖ **Pure Chocolate Mask:** Melt some dark chocolate in a bowl in the microwave. It's best to microwave it for 30 seconds to avoid burning the chocolate. Once the chocolate has melted, apply the melted mixture to your face and leave on for 30-40 minutes. Rinse your face after with luke warm water.

- ❖ **Chocolate Pack Mask:**

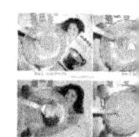

Mix thee tablespoons of coco powder, three tablespoons of honey, half a tablespoon of heavy cream, and half a tablespoon of oatmeal power until the mass is consistent. Apply on properly Cleansed face, gently massaging it so that oatmeal can exfoliate the dead skin cell. Leave it on for about 20 minutes and rinse off with cold water.

- ❖ **Chocolate, Honey, and Yogurt Mask:**

Blend cocoa powder with honey and yogurt. Cocoa powder can be difficult to blend, so be patient with this step. Keep mixing until mixture looks like melted chocolate. Clean your face with lukewarm water. Dab dry and then apply the mask evenly all over your face except the eye and lip areas. Relax for 15-20 minutes and let the mask do it's magic. Wash off with lukewarm water and dab dry.

❖ **Chocolate Brown Sugar Sea Salt Mask:**

Heat dark chocolate in a double boiler for about 3 minutes. Mix sea salt, brown sugar, and 2/3 of a cup milk in a bowl. Remove melted chocolate from heat.
Mix melted chocolate with salt/milk mixture.
Allow to cool.
Apply to face while cool but not hardened.
Leave on until it hardens.
Wash or chip off with mild cleanser and warm water.

❖ **Chocolate Oatmeal Mask:**

Mix all ingredients until mass in consistent.
Apply to face, gently massaging so oatmeal can start exfoliating the dead skin cell layer. Leave on for about 15-20 minutes
Rinse off with lukewarm water.

❖ **Chocolate, Avocado, Honey, and Oatmeal Face Mask:**

Mix a table spoon of coco powder, organic honey, smashed avocado, and three tablespoons of oatmeal together until mass is consistent. Apply on face, gently massaging so oatmeal can start exfoliating the dead skin cell layer. Leave on for 15-20 minutes then rinse off with lukewarm water.

Carrots

Carrots have many benefits for the body, for example, carrots are beneficial for the eyes since the Vitamin A they have helps the eyes to have good vision, increases immunity of the body, it can remove indigestible fibres for the body, and even prevent cancer from forming in the body. When it comes to skin benefits; carrots play a big role in that area as well. For example:

- **Skin Renewal:** Carrots contain Vitamin A, therefore, this help with tissue growth and skin renewal in the body. Vitamin A in carrots is in another form called beta-carotene
- **Prevents dryness:** this is due to carrots being rich in potassium.
- **Hydration:** Applying or drinking carrot juice hydrates skin.
- **Antioxidant:** Carrots contain a lot of antioxidants; therefore, it slows down the process of ageing, and fight free radicals which causes eczema, dermatitis, wrinkles, blemishes, scars and rashes.
- **UV ray protector:** Beta-carotene, antioxidants, and other caratenoids help defend the skin against UV rays and sun damage. Drinking carrot juice in the summer will give you skin a natural sun block to the sun rays.
- **Increases Elasticity:** Carrot contains Vitamin C, therefore, this help increase the production of collagen in the body; which gives the skin more elasticity. When elasticity of skin increases; the process of ageing wrinkles and lines is slowed down.

Recipes that Use Carrots

❖ **Carrot and Honey Face Mask:** Steam carrot until tender, leave to cool and mash in a bowl. Remove stone and skin from avocado, mash to a soft pulp and add to carrots. Add the honey and cream or yoghurt and mix well.
Apply in a thick layer to a thoroughly cleansed skin. Relax for 20 minutes and rinse off. Follow with a toner or splash of water and finish with a rich moisturiser. This mask can be kept covered and refrigerated, but should be used within a couple of days.

❖ **Carrot Face Mask:** Peal the carrots and steam until soft. Mash the carrots into a creamy consistency. Mix in 1 tbsp. of all natural honey. Stir in 1 tbsp. of olive oil. Squeeze a few drops of fresh lemon juice into the face mask mixture. Mix in enough mineral water to give the face mask a creamy consistency. The more lemon juice you added, the less water is needed for this step. Don't add too much, or your face mask will be runny. If you feel that the mixture does not need extra liquid, it is not necessary to include the water. Gently wash your face and neck with warm water and pat dry. Apply the mask evenly to your face and allow it to set for 15 minutes. Rinse your face and neck again with warm water and pat dry.

❖ **Carrot and Oatmeal mask:** extract the juice of a carrot and combine it with one tablespoon of raw honey. Once you have done this, add some blended oatmeal until it forms a good paste. Evenly smooth the mask mixture on your face, leave it on for fifteen and twenty minutes, before rinsing your face off with luke-warm or cold water.

❖ **De-ageing and wrinkle free Carrot Mask:** Steam thee carrots until they become soft, hence, after you have done this, blend the soft carrots with three teaspoons of raw honey and a teaspoon of glycerine. Apply it to face, leave it on for twenty minutes, before rinsing the mask of with luke-warm or cold water. Repeat this treatment two times a week to get the results you desire.

❖ **Carrot Mask for limp/sagging skin:** taker a soft steamed carrot and mash it with a teaspoon of extra virgin olive oil. Apply it face, leave it on for twenty minutes, message into face for three minutes, before rinsing the mask of with luke-warm or cold water.

❖ **Pimple and Mark Carrot Mask:** Mix one steamed soft carrot with a tablespoon of lemon or orange juice. Leave it on the face for twenty minutes before rinsing the mask of off with luke-warm or cold water.

❖ **Carrot and Avocado Mask:** Combine three soft and mashed carrots with one mashed avocado and four teaspoons of honey. Apply to face, leave it on for fifteen minutes, before rinsing mask off with luke-warm or cold water.

Coffee (Ground)

The caffeine contained in coffee is usually used in beauty skin care products in order to perk up and awaken skin. However, what the point of getting a little in a market product, were you can get the pure caffeine from ground coffee. The benefits ground coffee has on skin are:

- **Reduces Immflamation:** Caffeine contains anti-inflammatory properties, hence, this is useful for reducing immflamation on the skin as well as redness. Caffeine's inflammatory property is similar to aspirin.
- **Dark Eye Reducer:** Applying ground coffee under the eyes reduces puffiness which is associated with dark ring eyes. It reduces the amount of blood build up which is located under the eyes, hence, causes the dark shadows to appear.
- **Exfoliates Skin:** The extract of ground coffee, when applied on skin, removes dead skin cells, dirt, oils, and evens the skin surface. This leaves the skin soft and smooth.
- **Antioxidants:** Coffee contains antioxidants which help in riding the skin of free radicals, and stops the inner layer of the skin being damaged. This also helps with premature ageing, as well as ridding spots and pimples.
- **Rids Cellulite:** Ground coffee has been found to rid cellulite. Its able to do this be dehydrating the fat cells and energising them so the sodium and potassium component in them starts to vacate.
- **Tightens skin**: Coffee is especially good for tightening skin around the eyes and body.
- **Evens Skin**: Coffee constricts blood vessels in the skin, hence, this makes the blood vessels tighter and firmer. This leaves your skin youthful and smooth.

Recipes that Use Ground Coffee

1. **Exfoliation recipe:** Mix one cup of ground coffee, and four tablespoon of sweet almond oil or jojoba oil. Apply it to face, leave on for two-three minutes, before rinsing your face off with semi-warm water.
2. **Coffee Mask:** Mix three tablespoons of finely ground coffee with a small glass of milk. Mix together until it reaches a texture that's not too runny and not to thick. Apply to face, leave it on for 20 minutes, before rinsing the mask off with semi-warm water.
3. **Coffee Scrub:** Mix two tablespoons of ground coffee with one egg white and exfoliate your skin with it for two-three minutes. Once done, rinse face of with luke-warm or cold water.

Warning: Ground coffee can be very painful if it enters the eyes. If this happens, rinse the mask and ground coffee out of your eyes immediately with like warm or cold water. If you are unable to see after trying to rinse the ground coffee out of your eyes, call for help and contact emergency services.

Eggs

Egg: (White)

Egg white is very beneficial for skin since it contains nutrients which give the flowing benefits to the skin:

- **Tightening**: With the environment containing all types of free radicals our faces can easily lose tightness, become limp, and saggy. Usual use of egg whites will help tighten up skin; therefore, keeping the face youthful, closes pores, reducing lines, and gives your face a healthy glow.
- **Combat Oily Skin:** While egg white tightens the skin it also draws all the oils from your skin. Therefore, this leave your skin pore less and smooth.
- **Remove White heads:** The constant build up of debris and oil from the environment can create the well known skin problem called white heads. Therefore, egg white with abit of lemon helps clear white heads; well as nourish and heal skin.

Recipes that use Egg White

1. **Lemon and Lime mask (With Egg White):** This is the same as the Lemon and Lime mask. However, egg white is added so that it can absorb oils and debris; as well as the lemon and lime removing the first layer of skin. This mask will give you a new layer of soft skin followed by clean skin pores. For this mask you need to squeeze half a lemon and half a lime into a bowl before adding one egg white. You will need to separate the egg white from the egg yolk, before adding the egg white to the lemon and lime. Once the lemon, lime, and egg white are added, add ground oatmeal to the mask mixture to make it thicker. Once the mask has a thickened consistency, apply it to your face and leave it on for 40 minutes; or an hour. Once the time limit for the mask is over; rinse the mask off with cold water.

   Warning: For first time users of this mask it is important to know that once the mask is applied it will rather give a tingling sensation; or a semi burning sensation. This is the mask working into the pores and surface of the skin, however, if the sensation becomes too much for you, rinse your face of the mask as quickly as you can. To get used to the sensation of the mask its best that when you apply the mask, you leave it on longer than the time you left it last time. For example, if you leave the mask on your face, for the first time for ten minutes, the next time you used the same mask; you would leave the mask for fifteen minutes and so on. This helps your skin adjust to the sensations and after you have done this for a while you will only feel a tingling sensation and nothing more

   Warning Note: This mask is not advised for delicate skin since it can cause damage.

2. **Pure Egg White Mask:** For this mask you need only 1 egg white, therefore, you separate one egg yolk from the egg white, whisk the egg

white in a bowl; before applying it to your face. Leave the mask on for twenty to forty minutes before rinsing your face with cold water.

3. **Egg white Cleanser:** To a bowl add two table spoons of brown sugar, one egg white, and one teaspoon of lemon juice. Once you have done this; use your finger tips to exfoliate you skin in circular motion with the cleaner for fifteen minutes. Once you have done this, rinse your face with cold water.

4. **Turmeric Mask (With Egg White**): The egg will have the same benefits in each mask, however, along with the turmeric, you skin surface will be getting evened; while the egg rids of oils and debris in the pores. For this mask you would add one tablespoon of turmeric, once table spoon of rice flour, one table spoon of baking soda, one egg white, and one table spoon of milk. Mix this all together until you have a creamy thick consistency, and once done, apply the mask to the face and leave it on for forty minutes to an hour. Once you left it on for that long; rinse the mask off with cold water.

Warning: If this mask is left on for over an hour it can cause itching and extreme dryness. That's why it's very important for people who are using the mask for the first time to leave it on for twenty to fourty minutes before rinsing it off afterwards. If you suffer from dry skin, but still want the benefits of turmeric and egg white; add a little olive oil to the mix to even out the dryness and oiliness the foods will give to the skin.

Warning 2: If you are going to use eggs for any of your masks use organic eggs; since the battery farmed eggs usually contain chemicals which will absorb into your skin and cause damage.

Egg Yolk
Such benefits egg yolk can have on the skin are:
+ **Delays ageing:** Contains retinoids which gives skin a youthful glow. These retinoids are used in beauty products.
+ **Acne Treatment:** Their beneficial nutrient helps clear imperfections which acne causes.
+ **Moisturiser:** Egg yolk is usually used to moisturise skin. These types of mask are needed on people who suffer from dry skin.

Recipes that Use Egg Yolk
❖ **Egg Yolk Mask:** Separate an egg yolk from the white. Stir the yolk a little bit to break it up. If your skin is dry, add some olive oil and some warmed honey to the egg yolk. Use your fingers to apply it to your face and neck. Don't apply it on your eyes. Wait approximately 20 minutes and rinse it off using cool water.
❖ **Egg Yolk Mask 2:** Mix 1 tbsp. of honey, ½ tsp. of almond oil and 1 tbsp. of yogurt with 1 egg yolk.

Egg yolk mask with rich moisture: For skin that needs extra moisture; try this recipe for a face mask. Moisturize your skin with an egg yolk, avocado and mud facial mask. Simply mix 1 tbsp. of dry clay with 1 egg yolk and about ¼ cup of mashed avocado. You may also add witch hazel (use your own judgment on how much) for a smooth mixture. You will find that mud soaks up excess sebum, the avocado and egg yolk serve as moisturizers and the witch hazel will tone your skin.

Green Tea

Tea is an ancient herbal drink known for its stimulant qualities largely attributed to caffeine. In modern times, it also became touted as a health food allegedly helpful in preventing or ameliorating a variety of conditions, from heart disease and cancer, to gum disease, skin aging and weight loss.
(Taken from http://www.smartskincare.com)

Such benefits Green Tea has on the skin are:

- **Helps with dark eyes:** Applying moist teabag under the eyes for 5 minutes reduces puffiness and gives your eyes a more awakened and alert appearance.
- **Skin Cancer Protector:** Green tea extracts have been known to protect the skin against skin cancer.
- **Treatment for sun damage:** Green tea has been proven to treat sun damage on the skin. It's able to do this by extinguishing free radicals and decreasing inflammation.
- **De-ageing:** Green tea has been hypnotised to decrease the signs of aging, for example, this can be skin sagging, wrinkles. Although its not bee proven, green tea contains a lot of antioxidants and anti-inflammatory activities, hence, this can make that fact the green tea and decrease aging possible.

Recipes that Use Green Tea

- ❖ **Green Tea Anti-aging mask:** Break your fresh egg and place it into a glass container. Add three teaspoons matcha powdered green tea to the bowl along with three drops of lemon juice. Stir the ingredients well with a spoon. Slowly add honey to the mixture to form a thick paste.

- ❖ **Green Tea Mask:** Make a cup of green tea, with lots of tea. Twice as much loose tea as you'd normally use to drink or two teabags if you use tea bags. Leave the tea bags in for an hour, and if the tea is still warm (unlikely) chill it in the fridge until it's cool. Take it out, mix in the sugar and lemon juice, pat it onto your face and either use it as a face wash or (better) leave it on for 15 minutes.

Honey

Although bees can be the most irritating insects on the planet we still need them. There is even a theory that without bees out world and environment would perish; however, we won't be going over this subject; since it's another subject entirely. Bees have given us a natural gift and that gift is honey. Honey is one of the best ways to heal damaged skin and keep it youthful and young. The benefits of Honey on the skin include:

- **Moisturiser:** Since honey has Humectant properties (To produce moisture) this is excellent for people with dry skin. Honey helps to produce and retain moisture inside of the skin, therefore, it will leave your skin feeling hydrated and newly smooth.
- **Fights Acne:** Since Honey has microbial properties (Has the ability to inhibit the development of microbes and harmful microorganisms) it's especially good in fighting acne prone skin. This will end up giving you skin a clear non pimpled or freckled look.
- **De-ager:** The use of honey helps to rid winkles and other signs of ageing.
- **Antioxidant:** Honey is known to contain many antioxidants; therefore, this will help destroy free radicals, such as sunlight; which cause havoc on your skin. The antioxidant honey contains is called Myriad, therefore, these antioxidants neutralise free radials which are the cause of ageing.

Recipes that Use Honey

1. **Honey mask:** All you will need for this mask is pure honey. Therefore, apply honey to your face and leave it for fifteen minutes before rinsing your face with cold water. Doing this process two- three times a week will give your skin a real nourishing treatment.
2. **Honey, Cinnamon, and Nutmeg Scrub:** To a bowl add one tablespoon of honey, ground cinnamon, and ground nutmeg. Once in the shower massage the mixture into your face for one minute before rinsing the scrub off with cold water.
3. **Cucumber and Honey Treatment:** First you blend one cucumber in a blender before draining and collecting the juice. Once you have done this add two tablespoon of honey to the juice, pour the mixture into a bottle, and apply it to you face using cotton bud. Let the mixture air dry on your face before rinsing it off with cold water.

Note: You can keep the honey and cucumber mixture for up to a week, therefore, after that time period has finished; throw it out a make a new batch.

4. **Honey and Apple Treatment:** For this treatment what you need to do is blend one peeled apple (with core) with one tablespoon of honey; therefore, blend them until the mixture is smooth. Apply this to your face and leave it on for fifteen minutes before washing your face of the mask with cold water.
5. **Honey and Oat Face Scrub:** Mix one tablespoon of honey, finally ground almonds, dry oatmeal, and either lemon or yogurt; before massaging your

face with it. Once you have massaged your face with it for one-two minutes; rinse your face off with cold water.

Note: Your pores will get a lenitive cleaning. The reason this mask works so well is because almonds and oatmeal are the best sources for softening your skin and getting rid of dead skin.

6. **Honey Cleanser:** For this cleanser mix ¼ of honey, one tablespoon of liquid soap, and half a cup of glycerine. Apply this to your face using a face sponge and after exfoliating; rinse your face off with cold water.

7. **Honey Bath:** For your whole body to feel silky smooth add 1.4 cup of honey to your bath. This treatment is especially good for dry skin.

8. **Egg Yolk, Honey and Milk**

You can also create facial mask recipe by combining one egg yolk with 2 tbsp each of honey and milk together. After making the mask you can apply it smoothly on your skin and leave it for about 30 minutes before rinsing it off with water.

Warning: These honey recipes are not required for people who have allergic reactions to it. To get the same moisture effects you can rather use oil or avocados.

Lemon

Lemons are one of the sourest fruits ever found on the earth, therefore, the benefits of Lemon on the skin are:

- **Exfoliating:** Exfoliating with lemon preserves clear and youthful skin. The lemon is able to do this because its acids gently exfoliating the skin surface and pores.
- **Toner:** The use of Lemon juice shrinks pores, makes skin tight, and helps the skin to attain a nice glow.
- **Antiviral:** The presence of polyphenols in lemon oil can get rid of harmful viral bacteria which can cause cases such as cold sores.
- **Whitening**: For people who prefer a little whiting of the skin, lemon juice is an excellent source. Its use mostly to lighten freckles and dark patches which are usually located on the elbows or knees.
- **Environmental Protector:** Lemon contains the anti-oxidant Vitamin C which is good for combating sunlight, pollution, and daily stress.
- **Hydrates and Nourishes:** Due to the lemon containing Potassium, Magnesium; Vitamin B6, and folate; they help in the detoxifying, repairing, and renewal of the skin.
- **Minimises Wrinkles**: Vitamin C is responsible for the stimulation of collagen, therefore, this means that it can reduce and even clear winkles which are caused by our environment.

- **Cleans Pores**: For oily skin sufferers lemon juice is perfect for cleansing oily faces.
- **Lemon and Witch Hazel:** These two ingredients can help combat the most troublesome of problems. For example, the astringent effects of Lemon help to blemishes and excess sebum from acne.
- **Treatment for Dermatitis:** Dermatitis is a skin condition which can cause the person to have extremely dry and irritated skin with inflammation. Using lemon juice with Witch Hazel will help ease this condition. To find the recipe look at the treatment for dermatitis in the recipe section below.

Recipes that use Lemon

1. **Whitening Lemon Treatment:** Rub half a lemon on the dark areas of the skin to get results. The results can take a few months to show.
2. **Whiting Mask:** To a bowl add one tablespoon of lemon juice, tomato juice, cucumber juice and sandal wood pate. Once this has been mixed in apply to face and leave for fifteen minutes. Once the fifteen minutes are over; rinse face off with cold water.
3. **Lemon Cleanser:** To a glass of water squeeze half a lemon of juice, add cumber slices, cover the glass with a plate, and shake it before leaving it for five minutes. After the fives minutes have passed, dip a cotton bud into the water and wipe your face with the lemon mixture before rinsing you face with cold water.
4. **Lemon Cleanser 2:** To a bowl add two table spoons of brown sugar, one egg white, and one teaspoon of lemon juice. Once you have done this; use your finger tips to exfoliate you skin in a circular motion with the cleaner for fifteen minutes. Once you have done this, rinse your face off with cold water.
5. **Black Tea, Honey, and Lemon Mask:** Mix one tablespoon of black tea, honey, and lemon together, apply, and leave it on the face for twenty minutes. Once twenty minutes has passed, rinse the mask off with cold water.
6. **Wrinkle Fighting Mask:** For this mask all you need a milk and lemon juice. Apply this to the face for 10 minutes before rinsing your face off with cold water.
7. **Acne Cleanser:** Add Lemon juice to vinegar and use a cotton bud to wipe the mixture over the acne prone areas of your skin.
8. **Treatment for Dermatitis:** First soak gauze pads in a Witch Hazel solution before squeezing it and applying it over the affected areas of your skin. For itching relief this is where you add the lemon juice or lemon oil to the gauze pad before putting it on the affected area of the skin.
9. **Treatment for Puffy Eyes:** Apply Witch Hazel compresses to puffy eyes helps ease them and to stop dark circles and swelling. When you do this, leave them on for 5 minutes so they take effect.

10. Lemon and Lime Mask:

Warning: Excessive use of Lemon juice can cause skin damage due to the acidity of the lemon. It's important that you use any mask with Lemon once or twice a week to keep skin clean but not damage the skin overall.

Warning 2: Excessive use of Witch Hazel can also cause dryness, therefore, its best to use it in moderation. For people with delicate skin its best to dilute lemon with water before applying it to your face and sensitive skin.

Lime

Lime has similar properties to the skin benefits of Lemon; however, I wanted to do the benefits of lime on skin separately. One of the main benefits of Lime on skin is that it can help skin to be glowing and smooth even when you consume it. The paragraph below shows how lime is able to help skin from the inside to the outside

When your body processes nutrients, they oxidize. The results of this process are molecules that have an uneven number of electrons and are called free radicals. Free radicals start a chain reaction within your body, causing other molecules to oxidize. This entire process leads to a degradation of cells, which contributes to aging and damaged tissues. Certain vitamins, including vitamins A and C, act as antioxidants. Antioxidants absorb the brunt of the free radical chain reaction and allow them to be passed harmlessly from the body via the urine. According to the USDA National Nutrient database, 100 grams of raw lime contains 29.1mg vitamin C and 50 IU vitamin A. Adding limes to your diet can reduce free radical circulation within your body, leading to reduced tissue damage and fewer signs of aging, which in turn can lead to a brighter, more youthful complexion.

(Taken From http://www.livestrong.com)

Other benefits Lime has on skin are:

- **Anti-bacterial Agent:** The presence of bacteria on skin causes facial blemishes, inflammation, redness, soreness, and acne. Since lime contains natural antibiotic properties; it keeps acne bacterial growth at a low level.
- **Tightens Pores:** Lime juice contains astringent properties, therefore, astringents cause a temporary moment where the muscles suddenly contract. In commercial face products astringents are present, however, instead of use these products which can dry and damage skin; you can use lime which contains astringent properties to tighten skin. Other benefit lime has on the skin is that it can reduce oil production temporally in the skin and gives skin a bright clear completion.
- **Removes Dead Skin:** Lime juice contains citric acid, therefore, this is especially good for removing dead skin cells. This stops the dead skin from hiding you fresh new skin; giving you skin an overall new glow, stopping the pores from being clogged with dead skin, and decreases the chances of acne.

Recipes that use Lime

1. **Lime and Lemon Mask:** To a bowel mix the juice of half a lime, juice of half and Lemon and any other type of food which will give you skin benefits. Leave it on for about 20 minutes before rinsing you face off with cold water.

2. **Lime and Lemon Mask 2:** Bring to a boil a quarter cup of lemon peel, a quarter cup of lime peel, and lemon leaves. Steep for five minutes and add a tablespoon of lemon juice, two tablespoons of oats. Add a tablespoon of wheat germ. Let cool, and then apply on the face. Rinse off after 30 minutes.

3. **Honey Lime Mask:** Warm the honey and lime juice in a sauce pan over a very low heat, just until warm and soft. Move to a bowl and add the lavender. Smear over a clean face and neck, leaving on for twenty minutes. This is a great before bed mask. I like to wear it while soaking in a honey and milk bath for a double softening and cleansing skin treatment. This is a honey and lime heaven on earth pampering treatment. Relax, close your eyes and simmer in natural honey and citrus. Rinse well, splash the face with cool water and moisturize. This mask is especially good for balancing skin, therefore, it leave the skin not too oily and not too dry.

Milk

The main properties we know about milk is that it can help our bones and teeth to be strong; due to the high concentrations of calcium, Vitamin D, and Phosphorus that is in milk. However, milk can have beneficial effects on the skin as well, for example:

- **Cure for Acne:** Nutrients which are located in milk have been found by the University of Maryland Medical Centre to reduce the symptoms of acne.
- **De-ageing Treatment:** Since milk contains Vitamin A; its antioxidants helps to combat the signs of ageing. This benefit is also good for vegetarians; since they can have Vitamin B deficiencies from not eating meat.
- **Cure for Skin Problems:** Vitamin A, which is in milk, is known to bring the benefits of retinoids to the skin. Therefore, this means that it combats the pimple causing radicals of acne, unclogs pores, and calms down skin inflammation.
- **Soft Glowing skin:** I was known in the Egyptian times that Cleopatra took milk and Honey baths to keep are skin soft and glowing. The reason for this was because milk contains lactic acid which is good for the exfoliation and enzymes to sooth the skin.
- **Antioxidant:** Milk contains antioxidants which help combat environmental toxins which cause skin damage.

Recipes that use Milk

Warning for the First Four Recipes: The first four recipes listed below are mainly skin lightening mask recipes. If your aim is not to lighten your skin; do not use the first four recipes.

Warning 2: For anyone with milk or dairy product allergies; do not use these mask recipes.

1. Cow's Milk

Put some milk in a bowl whether it is a cow's milk or a goat's milk as both can lighten your skin. You can add buttermilk for added benefit of making your skin softer and smoother. This is an advice from the "1,001 Home Remedies and Natural Cures: From Your Kitchen and Garden." Place the bowl of milk in the microwave for at least 30 seconds to warm the milk.

Once the milk is warm soak a clean wash cloth into the milk. Make sure that the wash cloth should be fully saturated but not dripping. Gently massage the milk on a clean, dry part of the skin you want to lighten. If the wash cloth dries out, dip it again into the bowl to refresh its milk supply. It is best recommended if you have shower first before applying the milk so that you can be sure that your skin is well cleaned.

1. Egg Yolk, Honey and Milk

You can also create facial mask recipe by combining one egg yolk with 2 tbsp each of honey and milk together. After making the mask you can apply it smoothly on your skin and leave it for about 30 minutes before rinsing it off with water.

2. Lime Juice and Milk

Make a paste by combining milk and lime juice. Use one spoon of gram flour and mix it with 2 tablespoons of raw milk and a few drops of lime juice. After thoroughly combining the ingredients together, apply the mixture on your skin leaving it for 20 minutes before you rinse it with water. This paste can help lighten your skin and at the same time a good remedy for pigmented skin. This remedy can be used on a weekly basis.

3. Almonds and Milk

You can also soak some almonds in milk for a whole night then make a fine paste on the next morning which you can apply on the areas of the ski you want to lighten. Leave it on the skin for overnight and repeat the procedure everyday for two consecutive weeks.

4. Papaya and Milk

Mix 1 cup of papaya pulp ½ tsp each of honey, milk and rose water. Apply the mixture on your face and leave it for about 20 minutes before rinsing it off with water. This is a good remedy for a pale skin.

Squeeze the juice of a fresh lemon. Do not use frozen juice. Dip a cotton ball on the lemon juice and remove extra liquid to avoid getting it on your eyes during application. Lie down and place the wet cotton ball on the dark area you want to lighten up or simply pat the skin enough to wet it but don't let any juice come running. Let it sit in for about 20 minutes or may increase the time unless there is no pain or burning felt. Rinse thoroughly after the waiting time with cool water then pat dry.

5. Milk Rejuvenation for Skin Care
Blend together-

- 2 Tablespoon milk
- 1 Tablespoon turmeric powder
- 1/2 Tablespoon lemon

Mix ingredients & apply it to your face for younger & smoother looking skin.

Leave mixture on face 15-20 minutes. Rinse with tepid water. Pat dry.

6. Anti aging Milk & Honey Facial Mask
Mix together-

- 4 teaspoons of honey
- 3 teaspoons of milk

Apply this paste on your face as a facial mask. Leave it for 10-15 minutes and wash your face gently using warm water.

Repeating this skin care treatment every week will help keep your face young and glowing.

7. Milk Cleanser:
Dip a piece of cotton wool into a small bowl of already poured milk before smoothing it over you face. Leave the milk to dry on your skin before rinsing it off with luke warm water.

8. Soft and Smooth Skin Mask
Grind up 20g of Almond Nuts until there is a powder. Once you have done this stir and strain the almonds before adding milk to it and applying the mask on your face. Leave the mask to work on the skin for twenty minutes before rinsing your face with cold- Luke warm water.

9. Face Firmer Mask:
Boil milk until there is dry milk cream. Mix this cream with a little bit of rose water, apply to face, and leave it on for fifteen minutes, before rinsing it off with cold water.

Nutmeg

Nutmeg (a nut kernel) is similar to Cinnamon, hence, using them both can be a great way to clean your skin and make you entire countenance youthful. The benefits of Nutmeg on the skin are:

+ **Helps with Skin Problems:** Due to nutmegs antiseptic properties (which in turn kills bacteria); Nutmeg is very good for curing skin related problems. For example, this can be eczema, blackheads, rosacea, and acne
+ **Smoothes Skin**: Due to nutmegs exfoliating properties, it s also good for cleaning skin, removing dead skin cells, getting rid of oil, and overall refreshing the skin, hence, making the skin smooth. Nutmeg also contains essential oils which are very good for the skin.

+ **Anti-inflammatory**: with Nutmegs Anti-inflammatory properties, it is good for reducing inflammation and redness on the skin.

Recipes that Use Nutmeg

1. **Honey and Nutmeg Face Scrub (Acne Remedy Mask):** Mix on tablespoon of honey and one teaspoon of Nutmeg together. Apply to face, exfoliate for about 1-2 minutes, before rinsing your face off with cool or luke warm water. It can also be used as a face mask when left on for 30 minutes.

2. **Aid for Other Masks**: Nut can be used in conjunction to other face mask recipes to help the skin altogether. For example, the honey and cinnamon mask mixed with a little nutmeg will mean that are two exfoliates for the skin.

3. **Nutmeg and Milk Face Scrub**: Mix half a teaspoon of nutmeg with two tablespoons of milk. Apply to face, exfoliate for 1-2 minutes, before rinsing your face off with cold or luke warm water.

Warning: Nutmeg can dry skin your ski n if you don't moisturise you face with face cream afterwards. If you are allergic to nutmeg, avoid using it and use another exfoliate in this book which you won't receive allergic reactions from. People with sensitive skin should be careful when apply nutmeg, since it has a tingling feeling and depending on your skin, can cause inflammation. If immflamation occurs, rise immediately and use honey and yogurt rather as a mask or a face wash.

Oatmeal
Oatmeal is one of greatest foods to help treat skin. It has a lot of benefits and help combat all sorts of skin problems, hence, the benefits of oatmeal on skin are:

+ **Cleanses Skin:** Oatmeal, when use by itself as a typical scrub, exfoliates away dead skin cells, oil, dirt, and any other impurities on the skin. Because oatmeal has anti-inflammatory properties, it can be used for all skin types, including sensitive skin types. The reason oatmeal is better than soap is because it contains saponins; hence, this is a skin cleaning agent.

+ **Cures Skin Problems:** Cosmetic products can cause the skin to be irritated or inflamed. Therefore, oatmeal can be used to cleanse deep in the pores of the skin. Oatmeal is also known to treat rashes and other marks caused by plat or insect bites.

+ **Medicine for skin diseases**: People who suffer from acne, rosacea, chicken pox, or eczema can use oatmeal in their baths. This helps heal skin since it contains soothing properties. The use of oatmeal can also decrease the symptoms of ageing.

+ **Dry Skin treatment:** Using oatmeal on the skin can bring back the natural balance of moisture in the skin; hence, this can be used to reduce dry skin problems.

Recipes that use Oatmeal

1. **Base:** Oatmeal, once grounded using a blender, can be use in a range of masks to thicken the mixture; or already be used for it beneficial purposes.

2. **Basic Oatmeal Mask:** Take some ground oatmeal, add water, and mash it until it a soaked, squeeze the oatmeal so the juice falls on you other hand; before spreading it over your face. Use the soaked oatmeal to scrub you face for a minute before rinsing your face off with warm to cold water.

3. **Lemon and Lime Mask:** For this mask refer to the sections explaining the benefits of limes, lemons, and yogurt.

4. **Brown Sugar and Oatmeal Scrub:** To a small bowl add two tablespoon of ground oatmeal, brown sugar, and half an avocado. Mix it all together until it forms a paste. Massage this paste onto your wet skin for 2 minutes before rinsing the scrub off with warm to cold water.

5. **Oatmeal Bath:** While the water is running into the bathtub, add half a cup of ground oats, half a cup of almond milk, and some honey. Soak in the bath until done.

Olive Oil

Oils are very good for sorting dry skin problems. Such benefits olive oil can have on the skin are:

- **Anti-Inflammatory:** Olive oil contains nutrients such as Vitamin A and Vitamin E. It also contains an antioxidant called Hydroxytyrosol, hence, this antioxidant prevent free radical damage in the skin cells. This is why Olive oil is used by all skin types, especially those with severe dry skin.

- **Moisture:** Due to olive oil having tonnes of antioxidants, its very god for moisturising dry skin. From these antioxidants, they create a hydrophilic barrier, hence, spreading a protective coating over the skin. This protective coating keeps moisture inside of the skin pores.

- **Exfoliate:** Although some people think that using olive oil to exfoliate skin is the worst thing to do, olive oil is a very good natural exfoliate. It also good for softening and smoothing skin texture. This is due to new skin growth being made on the skin, while dead skin cells are exfoliated away.

- **Anti Ageing:** Vitamin E and Vitamin A is in Olive Oil; hence, this is good for healing damage from the sun, free radicals, and photo ageing. This helps make you skin look young, youthful, as well as rid the signs of ageing.

- **Rids Irritation**: Skin problems such as eczema or psoriasis can cause skin damage, redness, pain, and irritation. Olive oils antioxidants and healing properties help cool these skin problems down and over time can cure it fully.

Recipes that Use Olive Oil

1) **Olive Oil Face Wash**: Wash your face with luke warm water. Apply olive oil to your face and exfoliate your skin with it for about 2 minutes. Once done, rinse your face off with luke warm or cold water.
2) **Olive Oil, Honey, and Egg Mask:** Combine Egg white, one tablespoon of honey, and one tablespoon of olive oil together before applying it to your face. Leave it on your face for15 minutes daily before rinsing it off with luke warm to cold water.
3) **Olive Oil for Irritated Skin:** You can rather add a quarter cup of olive oil to you bath or apply the olive oil right on the irritated are of the skin.
4) **Make up Remover:** Although this book is for natural skin, some ladies will still love to wear makeup. For example, even though I always aim for natural clean skin, I still use mascara and lipstick. To remove make up dab a cotton ball with olive oil, place it on the area with make up for 30 seconds, before removing the

makeup away by sliding it over the area with makeup. You can also rinse you face after with water if you wish to clean your face even more from the makeup and oil.

5) **Olive Oil as an aid:** Olive oil can be used with other natural fruit and vegetables to benefit the skin. For example, the sugar and honey face scrub can also have olive oil added to it to rid dead skin cells and dirt even more.

6) **Moisturising Olive Oil Mask:** mix together one table spoon of olive and castor oil. Apply to face, leave it on for as long as you wish until you are satisfied, and then apply a hot wash cloth to your face for about a minute. Once you have done this, was your face off with luke warm to cold water.

Oranges

Although oranges don't seem to be a treatment fruit, at least it wasn't in my opinion until I tested it with a mask; it's still the best fruit use for natural beauty treatment. I add on a side note that this is good if you want a skin peel mask without the high acidity level lemon or lime juice would have, hence, it a very mild acidic fruit. The benefits of oranges on the skin are:

- **Skin Exfoliate:** Grounded Orange peels can be used as a scrub to clean and rid dead skin cells off the body. To create a scrub use orange peels which have been sun dried and grinded.
- **Gets rid of marks:** Due to sun damage, or even tanning, this causes skin to get dark marks, scars, and blemishes. Orange is a great solution for riding dark marks and blemishes that appear on the face.
- **Improves Overall Skin**: Because the orange contains Vitamin C, this helps with making your skin brighter, clearer, and dealing with uneven skin which is stopping your skin becoming even.
- **Pore Cleanser**: Oranges can help open the process and cleanse then from the inside. Therefore, by all the oils, dirt, and bacteria being cleaned, this gives the skin and face a bright, fresh, and newly clean appearance. This also helps combat acne that can affect the skin and damage it.
- **Anti-Ageing:** Oranges have the ability to restrain collagen in the skin. This stops signs of old ageing and saggy skin. Because oranges can combat early ageing signs, it can help rid wrinkles and softens the skin.

Recipes that Use Oranges

1. **Skin Glow Mask:** Mix sun dried ground orange peel with milk and ground oats. Apply to the face and leave for 30 minutes before rinsing your face off with water.

2. **Orange Peel Face Mask:** In the following box shows how a delightful orange peel mask can be made to clean and refresh the skin.

First of all you will need to clean the orange peel with some salt water so that all germs are removed from the fruit. Now put the peels in the blender and mash it up to make a thick sticky paste. Once the paste is ready, mix a tablespoon of yogurt to the paste. Add a few drops of lemon juice as well, and then add a teaspoon of honey or glycerine into the paste. Mix the paste thoroughly so as to allow all the ingredients to blend properly. Before you apply the pack, wash your face with warm water. Let the pores of your face open up by using some steam therapy. You can do this by leaning over a vaporizer or a jug of hot water. The steam will warm your face and open the skin pores. Now apply the pack evenly on your face and use a generous amount so that it is not too thin. The pack may sting a tiny bit, but it will be manageable. After this you must allow the pack to remain for about 45 minutes to one hour. Wash the pack when it's completely dry, or when one hour is complete, whichever happens faster. Wash the face pack with cold water and gently rub the pack off using your fingertips. Try to apply some bit of pressure with your fingertips so that all the dead skin and internal dirt can be removed simultaneously.

Taken From http://www.buzzle.com/articles/orange-benefits-for-skin.html

3. **Baking Soda and Orange Juice Mask:** Mix one tablespoon of orange juice with one tablespoon of baking soda. Apple to face let it set on your face for 20 minutes, and rinse face with water afterwards.

4. **Orange and Banana Face Mask:** Mix half a banana with one tablespoon of orange juice, and a tablespoon of honey. Apple the mask to the face let it set for fifteen minutes, before rinsing the mask off with cool water.

Pumpkin

Although some people think pumpkins are only used in Halloween, those critters with their creepy Halloween faces can also be used to benefit out skin. Hence, this reminds of the saying "Don't judge a book by its cover". Pumpkins can be found in organic markets, or even ordered via vegetable delivery companies. The benefits of Pumpkins on the skin are:

- **Brighten and Smooth Skin**: This is due to the fruit enzymes, and Alpha Hydroxyl Acids.
- **Decreases signs of Ageing**: This is able to be done by the Vitamin A, Vitamin, and C boosting collagen production in the skin.

- **Combats Acne**: Pumpkins contain alto of zinc, hence, this is great for those to suffer from acne. Zinc, when used on skin, helps control hormone levels, heals skin, and balances oil levels.

+ **Helps with Oily Skin**: Pumpkin Contains Vitamin E (Fatty Acids) which aids the protective function layer of the skin. This is great for oily skin, since it also regulates sebum which is naturally produced on our skin.

+ **Deeper Penetration**: Pumpkins can penetrate deeper into the skin than other types of fruits and vegetables.

+ **Medicine**: Pumpkin juice can be used to treat skin burns, abscess, pain, and cools down insect bites.

Recipes that use Pumpkins

- **Dark Eyes Fader Pumpkin Recipe**: Mix one tablespoon of pureed pumpkin, one teaspoon of honey, one teaspoon of lemon juice, and one teaspoon of vitamin E oil together. Apply to the areas where the eyes are dark, leave for thirty minutes, before rinsing off with luke warm to cold water.

- **Dry Skin Pumpkin Mask:** Mix one table spoon of yogurt with one tablespoon of pureed pumpkin together. Add to face, leave it on for thirty minutes to an hour, before rinsing your face off with luke warm or cold water.

- **Oily Skin Pumpkin Mask:** Mix together one tablespoon of pureed pumpkin and one table spoon of cider vinegar. Apply to face, leave it on for 30 minutes, before rinsing you face off with luke warm to cold water.

Rice Flour

I've always have used rise floor as a base to make of my other natural skin recipes, hence, I find it the best base not just for creating the right texture for a mask, but also the properties it gives to the skin. The benefits of rice flour on the skin are:

+ **Smoothes Skin**
+ **Brightens Skin (If this is your aim)**
+ **Absorbs oil and dirt from the skin.**
+ **Balances Skin pH**
+ **Anti ageing:** It helps rid wrinkles, pigmentation, as well as blemishes.
+ **Hydrates skin**
+ **fade dark spots and scars**
+ **Softens skin.**

Recipes that use Rice Flour

1. **Base:** Use with any other natural skin care ingredient (e.g.: juices peach, orange juice banana, etc) to benefits you skin and give you make a good texture so you can apply it onto you face.

2. **Rice Flour Mask**: Mix the rice flour with water (or natural skin care fruit or vegetable juices) until it's at the texture you prefer. Apply to face leave it on for 30 minutes, before rising it off with luke warm or cold water.

3. **Skin Cleaning Mask:** Mix once table spoon of rice flour with two tablespoons of yogurt. Apply to face, leave it on for 30-40 minutes, before rinsing your face with luke warm to cold water.

Sugar

Sugar is one of the best exfoliates for the skin. Its benefits are:

+ **Protects skin from toxins:** Sugar contains an acid called glycolic acid. This acid protects the skin from toxins as well as moisturises skin and keeps it healthy.

+ **Keeps Skin Healthy:** Sugar contains alpha hydroxyl acid, hence, this keeps skin healthy. This acid is used in chemical skin care products as well, however, getting it from the natural source is so much better for your skin

+ **Treatment for Acne:** Sugar can help with acne; hence, it cleanses the pores of trapped oil which can cause breakouts.

+ **Balances Oil in the skin**

+ **Rids blackheads and blemishes**

+ **Combats ageing**

+ **Brown Sugar:** If you prefer are more gentle exfoliate, it's best to use brown sugar. This is recommended for people with sensitive skin.

Recipes that use Sugar

1. **Sugar Cleanser:** To a bowl add two table spoons of brown sugar, one egg white, and one teaspoon of lemon juice. Once you have done this; use your finger tips to exfoliate you skin in circular motion with the cleaner for fifteen minutes. Once you have done this, rinse your face with cold water.

2. **Honey and sugar face scrub:** Mix together two tablespoon of honey with one tablespoon of sugar. Exfoliate the mixture with the scrub for three minutes before rinsing off with luke-warm or cold water.

   Warning: Excessive exfoliation of sugar scrubs damages skin. Use these recipes at least two times a week to even skin and remove dead skin cells. If you skin is smooth, it's not wise to use these scrubs after, since it can make skin uneven and damaged.

   Note: Sugar can also be used to rid dry skin and oil on feet, body, and hair.

Strawberry

Strawberries are one of the best known fruits for skin care. Apart from being delicious in salads, Eton mess, and benefiting the body inside and out, it's also good when it comes to natural regular maintenance care of your skin. The benefits of Strawberries are:

- **Exfoliate:** Since strawberries contains a high amount of alpha-hydroxyl acids, the fruit is very good for sloughing and removing dead skin cells of the surface of the skin.

- **Deep Cleanser:** Usually found in the beauty stores face cleansers and masks are salicylic acid. This naturally occurs in strawberries, hence, strawberries with its acid deeply clean into the pores of the skin to rid it of oil, dirt, free radicals and other factors from our environment. This also stops acne from occurring on the skin which is caused by those factors.

- **Sun Protection:** Strawberries contain Ellagic Acid. Therefore, this acid protects the skin from UV rays. This also helps with getting rid of pigmentation also caused by the sun rays.

- **Regenerate skin:** Strawberries contain a large amount of Vitamin C, hence, this help collagen production. Strawberries also contain a lot of antioxidants which altogether benefit the skin immensely. This also helps with ageing, hence, it will also anti-age you skin.

Recipes that Use Strawberries

1. **Strawberry Face Scrub:** Cut a strawberry in half and use it to exfoliate and rub all over your face. Leave the juice on for a few minutes before rinsing your face off with water (either luke warm or cold).

2. **Strawberry and Sugar Scrub:** Mix together two tablespoons of sugar with one tablespoon of olive oil and one big strawberry which has been mashed with a fork. Use it as a face scrub for 1-2 minutes, before rinsing your face off with cold or luke warm water.

3. **Strawberry and Yogurt Mask:** Mash four strawberries with a fork and mix them with one tablespoon of fresh cream, yogurt, and organic honey. Apply to face, leave it on for 10-20 minutes, before rinsing you face off with luke warm to cold water.

4. **Strawberry Acne Mask:** Combine five mashed strawberries, one tablespoon of honey, and some lemon juice together for applying it to the face. Leave it on for 10-20 minutes, before rinsing you face off with luke warm or cold water.

5. **Strawberries for Puffy Eyes:** Cut reasonable (medium) sized strawberry slices and place them over your eyes for ten minutes. If you like you can rather rinse the juice off with water, or apply eyes cream on the eyes so the juice can give the skin around the eyes more healing and its benefits.

6. **Strawberry Face Toner:** Mash some strawberries so they create a juice. Get a cotton pad, soak it with the juice, and apply it to your face. The juice can be kept and used for five days.

7. **Strawberries for Oily Skin:** Combine mashed strawberries and yogurt together before applying to the face. Leave the mask on for 10 minutes, before finally rinsing your face off with water.

8. **Aid:** Strawberry can be used in conjunction with other masks to benefit the skin.

Warning: For people who do not want to lighten their skin, don't use strawberry too much or in every mask.

Turmeric

Turmeric is a spice which is made from ground Curcuma (Or Curcumin) roots; therefore, their main uses are in curry powder. Known as one of the main traditional medicines in India and China; the best benefits of Turmeric is that it can slow down the development of cancers. The other benefits of Turmeric are that it can cure digestive problems, lower LDL cholesterol levels, lower blood pressure, and reduce acidity in the body. The benefits of turmeric for the skin are:

    ✦ **Even Skin Tone:** The main best property of Turmeric is that it evens skin which feels uneven, limp, or lumpy. This spice will lead your skin feeling plump, smooth, tight, and fresh. Indian brides would use turmeric as a paste to rub their body or face before they got married.

+ **Cancer Treatment:** Because Turmeric contains Cumin; a study has found that consuming this spice over a period of time can destroy the production of cancerous cells. The person cumin can kill oesophageal cancer cells are in 24hrs.

+ **Antiseptic:** Turmeric is a marvellous natural antiseptic and antimicrobial agent; therefore, it is used as medicine to treat cold sores, burns, boils, wounds, and cuts. Turmeric is also good for killing the bacteria that end up ion the pores of your skin and can cause acne.

+ **Pain Reliever:** Since Turmeric has Anti-inflammatory properties, it is used to treat arthritis and rheumatoid arthritis.

+ **Skin Problem Treatment:** Turmeric can help clear and sort out the following skin problems: blemishes, blackheads, dark spots, hyper-pigmentation, psoriasis, and eczema.

+ **Hair removal Cream:** Instead of going to the shop to buy all those expensive hair removal creams (Nair for example); use Turmeric mixed with warm castor oil to removes areas with unwanted hair.

+ **Hair Treatment:** To simulate the hair follicles and treat dandruff; you can use Turmeric. Other properties Turmeric is used in are hair dyes and colorants.

+ **Dry Skin treatment:** Although Turmeric is mostly used for oily skin (and people with combination skin think it will give them excessive dry skin), this is not true. Turmeric is also good for decreasing the chances of dry skin.

+ **De-ageing Treatment:** Because turmeric tightens skin elasticity, smoothes out wrinkles, and makes skin supple; this slows down the ageing process of human ageing.

+ **Reduce Pigmentation.**

+ **Detox:** Turmeric can detox the skins pores and Liver.

+ **Treatment for Depression.**

+ **Speeds up healing and remodelling of dry skin.**

Recipes that use Turmeric

❖ **Turmeric Mask for Oily Skin:** To a bowl add two to four tablespoons of turmeric, one table spoon of milk, one tablespoon of lemon juice, and one egg white until it makes a thick and non runny mixture. Before applying the mask, put on gloves to avoid staining of the hands and fingernails. Apply it to face for 30-45 minutes before rinsing it off with cold water. This mask balances oil levels again and even out the surface area of the skin.

Warning!: Use Gloves for the application of all turmeric masks; since turmeric as the unfortunate property of staining hands and fingernails with its colour. This can make your hands look unhygienic.

Turmeric for Hair Removal 1:

❖ Dissolve 5 tbsp. of table salt in 1/2 cup of boiling water. Cover and set aside.

❖ Pour 5 tbsp. of milk into a clean bowl. Add 6 tbsp. of turmeric powder and the salt solution. Stir will until it turns into a paste. The use of salt together with turmeric can soften and dissolve unwanted facial hair.

❖ Wash your face with warm water to help soften your skin and facial hair. Use a mild moisturizing soap and avoid using harsh antimicrobial soaps on your face to prevent your skin from getting dry.

❖ Apply the turmeric mixture generously to the areas of your face with unwanted facial hair. Massage in a circular motion for 15 to 20 minutes until it hardens and dries. Store any unused turmeric mixture in the fridge for the next day.

❖ Wash your face with cold water to remove the turmeric mixture. Do the above steps every day until you no longer see unwanted facial hair. It usually takes six to eight days before you can see results. You can also apply the mixture every day for several months to help make your facial hair grow slower, thinner and finer.

Turmeric for Hair Removal 2:

❖ Place 1 cup of chickpea flour in a small mixing bowl. Add 1/2 tsp. turmeric and then stir in a few drops of milk or cream. Stir until the mixture forms a smooth, thick paste.

❖ Spread a thin layer of the turmeric mixture on the area in the direction of hair growth. Allow the mixture to remain on the area for 20 to 25 minutes, or until the mixture is completely dry.

❖ Wipe the turmeric mixture off the area with a washcloth, rubbing gently opposite the area of skin growth. Remove any remaining mixture with warm water. Apply your favorite moisturizer to sooth the skin and replace lost moisture.

Turmeric for Hair Removal 3:

❖ Place 1 tbsp. chickpea flour in a cup. Add enough milk or water to form a thick paste.

❖ Stir in 1 tsp. cream or yogurt and a pinch of powdered turmeric. The mixture should be thick but spreadable.

❖ Wash your hands with soap and water so that any bacteria on your hands won't be transferred to your face. Cleanse your face, using a cleanser formulated for your skin type. Allow your face to air dry.

❖ Apply the chickpea flour paste over the facial area where you wish to remove hair. Smooth the mixture over the area in the direction of hair growth.

❖ Allow the mixture to dry completely, and then use a dry washcloth to scrub the area, working opposite the direction of hair growth.

❖ Pat your face dry with a soft towel, and then apply sweet almond oil or olive oil to the area to sooth the skin and replenish lost moisture.

Night Cream: Create a paste by mixing turmeric with milk or yogurt. Leave the turmeric on over night before rinsing it off with water in the morning.

Moisture cream: Adding a little Turmeric to your moisturizer product will help the benefits of turmeric work into the skin, face, and body.

Exfoliate and Skin Brightener Mask: Mix chickpea (or rice) flour with turmeric powder in equal proportions. To save time for future treatments, store the mixture in airtight bottle. Add raw or soy milk (or yogurt) to a teaspoon of chickpea/turmeric powder to make a paste. Apply evenly to the face and leave on for about 10-15 minutes. Wash the mask off with warm water.

Turmeric Mask to reduce Wrinkles: A mixture of milk and turmeric is good for fine lines and wrinkles. Mix turmeric powder and rice powder with raw milk and tomato juice, enough to form a paste, and apply to face and neck for 30 minutes. Rinse with lukewarm water. This mask also has the property of lightening skin.

Water
No matter what mask or scrub you use water will always be needed to wash of the mask; followed by the dirt, oil, and dead skin.

Why should hot water be used first?
Hot water should be used first because it helps open the pores of the skin; therefore, this allows the mask or scrub to work into the pores and clean away the free radicals which causes problems. Using a face steamer also does the same thing, however, if you don't have face steamer; you can just splash your face a few times with warm (or slightly hot water). If you use hot water to rinse the mask of your face you will only be leaving the pores open and allowing more dirt, oil, and free radicals to come and contaminate the pores. This is why it's very important that hot water is used first, and not to rinse, when you are about to apply a beauty skin treatment to your face.

Why should Cold Water/ Luke Warm be used last?
Cold, or lukewarm, water should be used last because it helps close the pores of the skin. Therefore, this means that the skin will be protected from the free radicals, dirt, and oil that would flow into the pores if they were left open. The closing of the skin pores also helps of the properties from the food used in the mask (or scrubs) to take effect and give the skin overall benefits.

Yogurt
Yogurt (Turkish meaning to curdle or thicken) is a creamy pudding like consistency which is create from the bacterial fermentation of milk or cream, therefore, it is made in many types of forms. For example, there arte fruit flavoured yogurts, plain yogurts, and yogurts with certain fat contents in. The production of yogurt requires their fermentation of milk or cream with active bacterial cultures. The first production of yogurt was in the year 5,000 BC where mammary animals are first domesticated. In the year 2000 BC yogurt was found to be used in cleaning

products and beauty lotions. In the industry; the bacterial cultures used are called Lactobacillus acidophilus, Lactobacillus Bulgaricus, and Streptococcus thermophlis. Apart from yogurt being used for savoury and sweet dishes; yogurt can also be used to benefit and revive damaged skin. The benefits of yogurt are:

- **Moisturiser:** Once of yogurts best properties is that it can bring a lot of moisture back to the face, therefore, it will leave you skin plump, supple, and wrinkle free. The lactic acid, a natural alpha hydroxy acid, in the yogurt helps smooth and exfoliate skin. Make sure to use a thick kind with active cultures for the ultimate beauty benefits.
- **Treatment for Sun Burn:** Since yogurt contains zinc; it is a perfect remedy for people who have suffered sun burns.
- **Acne Treatment:** Just the same as Turmeric; Yogurt contains antimicrobial and antiseptic properties. Therefore, this helps with fighting acne and skin breakouts.
- **Reduce Discoloration:** Although this property is not known, yogurt does contain small bleaching properties. Therefore, this helps combat discoloration, blotches, and spots of the skin caused mostly by the environment.
- **De-ageing Treatment:** Due to the lactic acid in yogurt, it helps to rid dead skin, tighten pores (which increase elasticity of skin, and gets rid of deep lines and wrinkles.

Recipes that Use Yogurt

- ❖ **Pure yogurt**: If you want to make pure yogurt (to save money or make sure pure substances are nutrition your skin) this is the recipe to do that. Firstly boil the milk before lowering the temperature to 45°C. Once you have done this; add one tablespoon of store brought variety to a small amount of milk before adding the rest of the milk to it. The mixture should be left at the temperature of 45°C for four to six hours before putting it in a refrigerator to set.
- ❖ **Pure Yogurt Mask**: Take some pure yogurt (I use mostly Greek yogurt), apply it to the face, and leave it on for twenty minutes before rinsing it off with cold water.
- ❖ **Lemon and Lime mask (With Yogurt):** This is the same as the Lemon and Lime mask. However, yogurt is added so that it can exfoliate dead skin cells away. This mask will give you a new layer of soft skin, added moisture so your skin is plump, and followed by clean skin pores. For this mask you need to squeeze half a lemon and half a lime into a bowl before adding a tablespoon of yogurt. Once the lemon, lime, and yogurt white are added, add ground oatmeal to the mask mixture to make it thicker. Once the mask has a thickened consistency, apply it to your face and leave it on for 40 minutes; or an hour. Once the time limit for the mask is over; rinse the mask off with cold water.

❖ **Yogurt and Lemon Face Mask:** Combine 2 tbsp. of plain yogurt with one to two drops of lemon juice. Be sure to use regular yogurt and avoid the fat-free or low-fat varieties. Apply the yogurt to your skin. Leave the mask on for at least 20 minutes. Wash your skin to remove the yogurt mask. You can add other natural ingredients to your mask if desired --- "Good Housekeeping" suggests combining 3 tsp. of honey and one peach or nectarine with 2 tbsp. of yogurt in its mask.

❖ **Sun burn Treatment:** Add a few drops of soothing chamomile essential oil to about a handful of organic yogurt. Rub the calming concoction over your sunburned skin and let it sit for 10 to 15 minutes before rinsing it off.

❖ **Acne Treatment:** Rub a dab of the yogurt into acne-prone areas. Let the yogurt work on the acne prone areas, and then rinse it off after 30 minutes.

❖ **Discoloration of Skin Treatment:** Rub a few tablespoons of yogurt mixed with a squeeze of lemon juice onto skin for 30 minutes, and then rinsing off the mixture. Repeat three times a week.

End

REFERCNES
Apples
(http://www.perfectskincareforyou.com, 2009-2012, An Apple a Day Keeps You Glowing All Day, http://www.perfectskincareforyou.com/2010/03/apple-day-keeps-you-glowing-all-day_04.html, Wednesday 19th December 2012)
(http://www.leonoredvorkin.com, 2012, The Benefits of Apples, http://www.leonoredvorkin.com/henu/benapples.php, Wednesday 19th December 2012)
(http://www.epicbeautyguide.com, 2012, DIY Mask for Smooth Moist Skin, http://www.epicbeautyguide.com/2010/09/diy-apple-mask-for-smooth-moist-skin/, Wednesday 19th December 2012)
(http://www.livestrong.com, 2012, How To Make An Apple Facial Mask, http://www.livestrong.com/article/181515-how-to-make-an-apple-facial-mask/, Wednesday 19th December 2012)
Avocados
(www.3fatchicks.com, 2008, 5 Beauty Benefits of Avocado, http://www.3fatchicks.com/5-beauty-benefits-of-avocados/, Wednesday 9th January 2013)

(homecooking.about.com, 2013, Avocado Facts,
http://homecooking.about.com/cs/foodfactsheets/p/avocado_pro.htm,
Wednesday 9th January 2013)

(www.healinglifestyles.com, 2013 Avocado Recipes,
http://www.healinglifestyles.com/index.php/avocadorec10, Thursday 10th
January 2013)

(www.skincare.about.com, 2013, Avocado Citrus Mask for Dehydrated Skin,
http://skincare.about.com/od/spa/a/AvocadoCitrusFacialMasque.htm,
Thursday 10th January 2013)

Banana

(www.hort.purdue.edu, 2013, Banana,
http://www.hort.purdue.edu/newcrop/morton/banana.html#Origin%20and%20
Distribution, Thursday 10th January 2013)

(newkiddy.blogspot.co.uk, 2013, Amazing Benefits of Bananas,
http://newkiddy.blogspot.co.uk/2012/04/benefits-of-bananas.html, Thursday
10th January 2013)

(beauty.about.com, 2013, Banana Mask for Oily Skin,
http://beauty.about.com/od/fragrance/r/bananamask.htm, Thursday 10th
January 2013

(www.ilovenaturalskincare.com, 2012, Banana Mask Recipes,
http://www.ilovenaturalskincare.com/banana-mask.html, Friday 11th January
2013)

Baking Soda

(www.ilovenaturalskincare.com, 2011, Homemade Facial Scrub Recipes,
http://www.ilovenaturalskincare.com/facial-scrub-
recipes.html#bakingSodaScrubs, Thursday 31st January 2013)

(www.livestrong.com, 2013, Health Benefits of Bicarbonate Soda,
http://www.livestrong.com/article/110287-health-benefits-bicarbonate-soda/,
Thursday 31st January 2013)

(www.healthguidance.org, 2013, Health benefits of Baking Soda,
http://www.healthguidance.org/entry/15156/1/Health-Benefits-of-Baking-
Soda.html, Thursday 31st January 2013)

(www.makeupbeautyetc.com, 2013, Baking Soda Benefits, www.makeupbeautyetc.com, Thursday 31st January 2013)
Cucumber
(www.disabled-world.com, 2013, Cucumber Benefits for Great Skin and Eyes, http://www.disabled-world.com/artman/publish/cucumber_benefits.shtml, Friday 11th January 2013)
(Natural-homeremedies-for-life.com/, 2009-2013, Cucumber Mask Recipe, http://www.natural-homeremedies-for-life.com/cucumber-mask.html, Wednesday 16th January 2013)
Coffee (Ground)
(http://www.livestrong.com, 2013, What are the benefits of coffee for skin care?, http://www.livestrong.com/article/98727-benefits-coffee-skin-care/, Tuesday 22nd January 2013)
(http://ezinearticles.com, 2013, How About Some Coffee With you Skin Care?, http://ezinearticles.com/?How-About-Some-Coffee-With-Your-Skin-Care?&id=657018, Tuesday 22nd January 2013)
(www.ehow.com, 1999-2013, What are the Benefits of Coffee Scrub, www.ehow.com/list_7216438_benefits-coffee-scrub_.html, Tuesday 22nd January 2013)
(http://lifehackery.com, 2009, 11 Good Reasons Why Coffee Grounds are Worth Keeping, http://lifehackery.com/2008/08/21/home-7/, Tuesday 22nd January 2013)
(http://www.purefectyourskin.com, 2013, Coffee Face Mask Recipe for natural Skin, http://www.purefectyourskin.com/coffee-face-mask-recipe.html, Tuesday 22nd January 2013)
(http://www.purefectyourskin.com, 2013, Ground Coffee, http://www.purefectyourskin.com/coffee.html, Tuesday 22nd January 2013)
Cinnamon
(www.wisegeek.com, 2003-2012, What Exactly is Cinnamon?, http://www.wisegeek.com/what-exactly-is-cinnamon.htm, Friday 19th October 2012)

(www.livestrong.com, 2012, Benefits of Ground Cinnamon, http://www.livestrong.com/article/91597-benefits-ground-cinnamon-skin/, Friday 9th November 2012)

Castor Oil

(http://skinverse.com, 2013, Castor Oil for Beautiful Skin, skinverse.com/castor-oils-many-uses-for-beautiful-skin-and-hair.html#Castoroilacne, Wednesday 28th August 2013)

Milk

(http://www.livestrong.com, 2012, The Benefits of Milk For Skin, http://www.livestrong.com/article/466686-the-benefits-of-milk-for-skin/, Thursday 13th December 2012)

(http://www.fitday.com, 2000-2011, 6 Health Benefits of Milk, http://www.fitday.com/fitness-articles/nutrition/healthy-eating/6-health-benefits-of-milk.html, Thursday 13th December 2012)

(http://skinlighteningadvice.com, 2012, Skin Lighting with Milk Using Five Recipes, http://skinlightening.com/skin-lightening-with-milk-using-5-recipes/, Thursday 13th December 2012)

(http://www.anti-aging-skin-care-illusions.com, 2012, Natural Skin Care Recipes Using Milk, http://www.anti-aging-skin-care-illusions.com/natural-skin-care-recipes-using-milk.html, Thursday 13th December 2012)

(http://www.beautyandgroomingtips.com, 2006, Milk for Health and Beauty, http://www.beautyandgroomingtips.com/2006/04/milk-for-health-and-beauty.html, Thursday 13th December 2012)

Chocolate

---

http://www.wiseshe.com, 2012, Good Skin Care With Chocolate, http://www.wiseshe.com/2011/01/good-skin-care-with-chocolate-mask-and-benefit-of-chocolate-in-skin-care.html, Monday 10th December 2012)

(http://beautytips.ygoy.com, 2012, 10 Benefits of Chocolate, http://beautytips.ygoy.com/2008/09/29/0-benefits-of-chocolate-skin-care/, Monday 10th December 2012)

(http://www.thedailybeast.com, 2012, 11 Reasons Chocolate is Good for you Health, http://www.thedailybeast.com/articles/2012/03/28/11-reasons-chocolate-is-good-for-your-health.html, Monday 10th December 2012)

(http://dyingforchocolate.blogspot.co.uk, 2012, 5 DIY Chocolate Face Mask Recipes, http://dyingforchocolate.blogspot.co.uk/2012/08/tuesday-tips-5-diy-chocolate-face-mask.html, Monday 10th December 2012)

Carrots

(http://www.ehow.com, 1999-2013, How to make a carrot mask,http://www.ehow.com/how_2108020_make-carrot-face-mask.html, Monday 11th February 2013)

(http://www.lilianmay.co.uk, 2013, Recipe: Carrot and Honey Mask, http://www.lilianmay.co.uk/2011/08/recipe-carrot-and-honey-face-mask.html, Monday 11th February 2013)

(http://suvens.com, 2013, Carrot Face Mask for Recipes for Glowing Skin, http://suvens.com/beauty/homemade-face-masks/carrot-face-mask-recipes-for-glowing-skin/, Monday 11th February 2013)

Egg White

(www.livestrong.com, 2011, Benefits of Egg White, http://www.livestrong.com/article/89036-benefits-egg-white-face/, Wednesday 14th November 2012)

Egg Yolk

(http://www.ehow.com, 1999-2013, How to make an egg yolk face mask, http://www.ehow.com/how_4471439_make-egg-yolk-face-mask.html, Monday 11th February 2013)

(http://benefitof.ne, 2013, Benefits of Egg Yolk on face, http://benefitof.net/benefits-of-egg-yolk-on-face/, Monday 11th February 2013)

Green Tea

(www.smartskincare.com, 1999-2012, What Green tea can and cannot do for you skin), http://www.smartskincare.com/treatments/topical/greentea.html, Monday 11th February 2013) (http://lifeandbows.com/, 2012, Homemade Green Tea Face Mask, http://lifeandbows.com/homemade-green-tea-face-mask/, Monday 11th February 2012)

(http://www.beauty-and-the-bath.com, 2005-2012, Green Tea Mask, http://www.beauty-and-the-bath.com/green-tea-mask.html, Monday 11th February 2013)

Honey

(www.crunchybetty.com, 2010, Food on your face: Honey, http://www.crunchybetty.com/food-on-your-face-honey, Friday 16th November 2012)

(askville.amazon.com, 2006-2012, Why is Honey good for the skin?, http://askville.amazon.com/honey-skin/AnswerViewer.do?requestId=42731755, Friday 16th November 2012)

(learnerview.ofsted.gov.uk, 2006-2012, Natural Skin Care with Honey, http://www.benefits-of-honey.com/honey-and-skin-care.html, Friday 16th November 2012)

Lemon

(www.infobarrel.com, 2008-2012, Does Lemon Juice Lighten Skin?, http://www.infobarrel.com/Does_Lemon_Juice_Lighten_Skin, Wednesday 14th November 2012)

(http://www.beautifulskincareblog.com, 2011, 7 Benefits of Lemon for your skin, http://www.beautifulskincareblog.com/7-benefits-of-lemon-for-your-skin/, Thursday 15th November 2012)

(http://www.livestrong.com, 2012, Lemon Oil and Witch Hazel for the face, http://www.livestrong.com/article/528719-lemon-oil-witch-hazel-for-the-face/, Thursday 15th November 2012)

(http://blog.naturalhealthyconcepts.com, 2012, Can Lemon Juice really help Lighten you Skin?, http://blog.naturalhealthyconcepts.com/2012/05/09/can-lemon-juice-really-help-lighten-your-skin-2/, Thursday 15th November 2012)

(www.livestrong.com, 2012, The Benefits of Lemon on Skin, http://www.livestrong.com/article/101061-benefits-lemon-oil-skin/, Friday 16th November 2012)

Lime

(http://www.livestrong.com, 2012, The Benefits of Lime For The Face, http://www.livestrong.com/article/528332-the-benefits-of-lime-for-the-face/, Friday 14th December 2012)
(http://www.pioneerthinking.com, 1999-2012, Homemade Facial Mask Recipes, http://www.pioneerthinking.com/beauty/skin/facials-scrubs/sw_homefacials.html, Friday 14th December 2012)
(http://homemadefacemaskrecipes.blogspot.co.uk, 2010, Honey Lime Face Mask To Balance Skin, http://homemadefacemaskrecipes.blogspot.co.uk/2012/04/honey-lime-face-mask-to-balance-skin.html, Friday 14th December 2012)
Nutmeg
(www.fitday.com, 2000-2013, 7 Health Benefits of Nutmeg, www.fitday.com/fitness-articles/nutrition/healthy-eating/7-health-benefits-nutmeg-provides.html, Monday 2dn September 2013)
(http://www.care2.com, 2013, 8 Amazing Health Benefits of Nutmeg, http://www.care2.com/greenliving/8-amazing-health-benefits-of-nutmeg.html, Monday 2nd September 2013)
(http://www.satvikshop.com, Nutmeg, N/blog/herbs-knowledge-base/nutmeg, Monday 2nd September 2013)
(http://www.peachesandblush.com, 2012, How to get clearer skin with Nutmeg, http://www.peachesandblush.com/2012/01/how-to-get-clearer-skin-with-nutmeg.html, Monday 2nd September 2013)
(http://www.lizmarieblog.com, 2011, Honey Nutmeg Face Mask, http://www.lizmarieblog.com/2011/11/honey-nutmeg-face-mask/, Monday 2nd September 2013)
Oatmeal
(www.naturalnews.com, 2008, Oats for Beautiful Skin, http://www.naturalnews.com/024319_skin_natural_smooth.html, Wednesday 20th March 2013)
(http://hildablue.com, 2013, Ode to Oats, http://hildablue.com/2011/11/27/ode-to-oats-5-ways-to-benefit-from-oatmeal-in-skin-care/, Wednesday 20th March 2013)

(http://benefitof.net, 2013, Benefits of Oatmeal on Skin, http://benefitof.net/benefits-of-oatmeal-on-skin/, Wednesday 20th March 2013)

Olive Oil

(http://comluv.com, 2013, Benefits of Olive Oil, http://comluv.com/benefits-of-olive-oil-on-skin-health/, Wednesday 28th August 2013,)

(http://www.livestrong.com, 2013, The benefits of olive oil in skin care, http://www.livestrong.com/article/255334-the-benefits-of-olive-oil-in-skin-care/, Wednesday 28th August 2013)

(http://answers.yahoo.com, 2013, Benefits of Olive Oil on Skin?, http://answers.yahoo.com/question/index?qid=20100817135837AAFMp96, Wednesday 28th August 2013)

Oranges

(http://www.beautybets.com, 2010, Baking Soda and Orange Mask, http://www.beautybets.com/2010/06/diy-baking-soda-face-mask/, Saturday 6th April 2013)

(http://khoobsurati.com, 2011, Benefits of Orange for Hair and Skin, http://khoobsurati.com/blog/benefits-of-orange-for-hair-and-skin.html, Saturday 6th April 2013)

(http://www.buzzle.com 2000-2012, 2013, Orange Benefits for skin, http://www.buzzle.com/articles/orange-benefits-for-skin.html, Saturday 6th April 2013)

(http://www.perfectskincareforyou.com, 2009-2013, Benefits of Orange on Skin, http://www.perfectskincareforyou.com/2010/03/benefits-of-orange-on-skin.html, Saturday 6th April 2013)

Pumpkins

(http://www.stylecraze.com, 2013, 15 Best Benefits of Pumpkin Juice for Skin, Hair, and Health, http://www.stylecraze.com/articles/benefits-of-pumpkin-juice-for-skin-hair-and-health/, Tuesday 20th August 2013.

(http://blackhairmedia.com, 2013, The Hair and Skin Benefits of Pumpkin, http://blackhairmedia.com/hair-care/the-hair-and-skin-benefits-of-pumpkin/, Wednesday 28th August 2013)

(http://www.dermalinstitute.com, 2012, The Benefits of Pumpkin Ingredients on the Skin, http://www.dermalinstitute.com/us/news/?p=1638, Wednesday 28th August 2013)
Rice Flour
(http://beforeitsnews.com, 2013, Massive Benefits of Rice Flour, http://beforeitsnews.com/health/2013/05/the-massive-benefits-of-rice-flour-2485958.html, Wednesday 28th August 2013)
(http://www.bubzbeauty.com, 2013, DIY Skin Rescue Remedy, http://www.bubzbeauty.com/bubbi-likes/298-diy-skin-rescue-remedy.html, Wednesday 28th August 2013)
Sugar
(http://skincare.lovetoknow.com, 2006-2013, Benefits of Brown Sugar, http://skincare.lovetoknow.com/Benefits_of_Brown_Sugar_Scrub#, Monday 2nd September 2013)
(http://ellasbeautytips.wordpress.com, 2013, Sugar Benefits on Skin, http://ellasbeautytips.wordpress.com/tag/sugar-benefits-on-skin/, Monday 2nd September 2013)
Strawberries
(http://skincaredirect.org, 2013, Skin Care with Strawberries, http://skincaredirect.org/skin-care-with-strawberries.html, Monday 2nd September 2013)
(http://beautybanter.com, 2013, Strawberry Honey Acne Mask, http://beautybanter.com/diy-strawberry-acne-mask, Monday 2nd September 2013)
(http://foodtofitness.com, 2013, Health Benefits of Strawberry, http://foodtofitness.com/health-benefits-of-strawberry/, Monday 2nd September 2013)
(http://www.care2.com, 2013, 8 Beauty Tips with Strawberries, http://www.care2.com/greenliving/strawberries-kitchen-cupboard-beauty.html?page=2M, Monday 2nd September 2013)

(http://prakritiherbals.wordpress.com, 2013, Glow food for the skin- yummy Strawberries, http://prakritiherbals.wordpress.com/2012/04/13/glow-food-for-the-skin-yummy-strawberries/, Monday 2nd September 2013)

Turmeric

(http://www.bookmydoctor.com, 2011, Benefits of Turmeric, http://www.bookmydoctor.com/health-article/health-benefits-of-turmeric-198/, Thursday 6th December 2012)

(http://articles.timesofindia.indiatimes.com, 2012, Try Turmeric for Supple Skin, http://articles.timesofindia.indiatimes.com/2012-12-04/beauty/28363267_1_turmeric-skin-colour-indian-brides, Thursday 6th December 2012)

(http://www.livestrong.com/article, 2012, Homemade Facial Removal, http://www.livestrong.com/article/206884-homemade-facial-hair-removal/, Thursday 6th December 2012)

(http://www.livestrong.com, 2012, How to use Turmeric for Hair Removal, http://www.livestrong.com/article/218480-how-to-use-tumeric-for-hair-removal/, Thursday 6th December 2012)

(http://multiculturalbeauty.about.com, 2012, Turmeric for Beauty?, http://multiculturalbeauty.about.com/od/Skincare/a/Turmeric-For-Beauty.htm, Thursday 6th December 2012)

(http://www.healthdiaries.com, 2005-2012, 20 Health Benefits of Turmeric, http://www.healthdiaries.com/eatthis/20-health-benefits-of-turmeric.html, Thursday 6th December 2012)

Yogurt

(http://www.culturesforhealth.com, 2012, what is Yogurt?, http://www.culturesforhealth.com/what-is-yogurt-history, Thursday 6th December 2012)

(http://www.wisegeek.com, 2003-2012, What is Yogurt?, http://www.wisegeek.com/what-is-yogurt.htm, Thursday 6th December 2012)

(http://www.livestrong.com, 2012, The Skin Benefits of Lemons and Yogurt, http://www.livestrong.com/article/513736-the-skin-benefits-of-lemons-and-yogurt/, Thursday 6th December 2012)

(http://www.organicauthority.com, 2010, 5 ways Yogurt keeps skin Glowing and Gorgeous, http://www.organicauthority.com/delicious-beauty/5-skin-rejuvenating-treatments-using-yogurt.html, Thursday 6th December 2012)